PHARMACOTHERAPEUTICS OF STEROIDS IN DENTISTRY

AF528711

Authors

DR. ANAND CHOUDHARY (MDS)

PROFESSOR, DEPT. OF ORAL MEDICINE AND RADIOLOGY

HAZARIBAGH COLLEGE OF DENTAL SCIENCES AND HOSPITAL

DR. PALLAVI KESARWANI (MDS)

ORAL PATHOLOGIST

DENTAL OFFICER

JHARKHAND HEALTH SERVICE

BOOK RIVERS
WE CREATE READERS

Copyright©: Authors

All Rights Reserved

No part of this publication may be reproduced, transmitted or stored in a retrieval system, in any form or by any means, electronic, mechanical, photocopying recording or otherwise, without the prior permission of the author.

Website: www.bookrivers.com

Email: publish@bookrivers.com

Mobile: +91-9695375469

Place: Lucknow

Year: 2020

Address: C-1484, Indira nagar, lucknow 226016 near C-block churaha.

MRP: 299/-

ISBN: 978-93-90548-72-9

Acknowledgements

We thank almighty GOD

We would like to thank everyone who has taught us to gain knowledge during our academic pursuit. Their tireless effort for academic excellence and professional insight were a source of constant encouragement and inspiration. We are honored to have them as our teachers.

Writing a book is harder than we thought and more rewarding than we could have ever imagined. None of this would have been possible without our mutual co-operation and hard work .

On a personal note, we are eternally thankful to our parents and our daughters. Their patience and unquestioning co-operation have meant a lot to us.

At last we are also thankful to our students whose constant inspiration and support have made this work possible.

Preface

Corticosteroids, since their introduction in the 1940s, have become one of the most widely prescribed class of drugs. They belong to a class of chemicals that includes steroid hormones that are produced naturally in the adrenal cortex of vertebrates and analogous to those that is synthesized in laboratories. They have been used extensively in managing many oral diseases, due to their excellent anti-inflammatory and immuno-modulatory effects. Person on steroid therapy have altered responses to infection and wound healing. However, considering their potential and significant side-effects, they are sometimes termed as the "double-edged sword" in the field of medicine. Their successful use depends upon the comprehension of the disease process. This includes an appropriate diagnosis, a clear view of the desirable treatment outcome and understanding of whether the treatment is aimed at the management of a chronic disease or enhanced resolution of a short-term condition. The possible beneficial effects of systemic corticosteroids must be weighed against probable risks. This book is aimed at highlighting the pharmacology of steroids and its applications in the treatment of various oral conditions and lesions, and deriving a certain protocol for the same.

Dr. Anand Choudhary MDS

Dr. Pallavi Kesarwani MDS

CONTENTS

1.	Introduction	7
2.	History	10
3.	Anatomy of Adrenal Glands	13
4.	Hormones of Adrenal Cortex	16
5.	Regulation of ACTH	22
6.	Metabolism and excretion of Adrenal corticoids	32
7.	Glucocorticoids	35
	- Pharmacological Actions	35
	-Adverse reactions	57
	-Drug interactions	76
	- Precautions during glucocorticoid therapy	77
	- Contraindications	78
	- Preparations and doses	78
	- Uses in dentistry	101
8.	Conclusion	185
9.	References	186

INTRODUCTION

Corticosteroids are medicines that are similar to the natural hormone cortisone and belong to the family of drugs called steroids.

A hormone is a chemical substance that is secreted into the body fluids by one cell or a group of cells and has a physiological effect on other cells of the body. Chemically, hormones can be of 3 basic types steroid hormones; derivatives of amino acid tyrosine, and proteins or peptides.

Steroid hormones have a chemical structure similar to that of cholesterol, and in most cases are derived from cholesterol itself. Different steroid hormones are secreted by adrenal cortex, ovaries, testes and placenta.

The two major types of adrenocortical hormones are the mineralocorticoids and the glucocorticoids secreted by the adrenal cortex.

The mineralocorticoids have been called so because of their effects on the electrolytes of the extra cellular fluid - sodium and potassium in particular.

Glucocorticoids are a group of adrenal corticosteroids, which originally were considered to be concerned with influencing the blood sugar level; glycogen storage and carbohydrate turn over. However, both glucocorticoids and mineralocorticoids possess both types of actions to greater or lesser extent .

Adrenocorticoids exert a wide variety of physiological effects and pharmacological actions in the body. They enable the organism to resist various types of noxious stimuli and environmental changes termed 'stress'. The adrenal cortex is the organ, par excellence, of survival. When exposed to stress, an adrenalectomized animal dies quickly unless pretreated with corticosteroids.

Over 40 steroid hormones have been isolated from extracts of the adrenal cortex, but only about 7 have appreciable activity.

In addition to these naturally occurring compounds, several new steroids with glucocorticoid activity have been synthesized.

These agents are employed both for replacement therapy and for the treatment of diverse non-endocrine diseases. Corticosteroids exert profound effect on almost every organ system. Because of these diverse actions, they are among the most widely used class of drugs.

Corticosteroids and their synthetic analogues are commonly used for their potent anti inflammatory and immunosuppressive property in the treatment of a variety of conditions characterized by chronic inflammation and immune phenomena. When used properly, corticosteroids are a valuable asset.

As a consequence of their pleiotropic effects, the clinical use of and withdrawal of corticosteroids are complicated by a number of serious side effects, some of which are life threatening. Therefore, the decision to institute therapy with corticosteroids always requires a careful consideration of the relative risks and benefits in each patient.

Since a dichotomy, cannot be made between the mouth and the rest of the body, many systemic diseases manifest and produce oral lesions. The use of corticosteroids in either systemic or topical form, to treat such lesions by the practicing dentist has increased recently.

Dentistry, in the past few decades, has reached new heights. With the increasing awareness of the general public towards oral and dental diseases, and the general physician referring many patients for expert care, the number of medically compromised patients visiting the dentist has enormously increased.

Patients who have undergone therapy with glucocorticoids present unique problems for the dentist. Persons currently receiving steroid therapy have an altered response to infection and wound healing. More important is that the patients who are taking or have taken glucocorticoids have high risk of developing acute adrenal insufficiency when placed in a stressful situation.

The dentists must have correct knowledge of the dose, frequency and duration of steroid being prescribed by the physician, to enable the dentist to assess the need for supplementation of the same during the dental procedure. The dentist should also have thorough knowledge of the safe and effective use of these drugs for dental related therapy.

*

HISTORY

Addison (1849) first appreciated the clinical importance of the adrenal glands and described fatal outcomes in patients with adrenal destruction during a presentation to the South London Medical Society.

Brown sequard (1856) demonstrated that bilateral adrenalectomy was fatal in laboratory animals. It was later shown that the adrenal cortex, rather than the medulla, was essential for survival in these experiments. Further studies demonstrated that the adrenal cortex regulated both carbohydrate metabolism, and fluid and electrolyte balance.

Efforts by a number of investigators ultimately led to the isolation and characterization of the various adrenocorticosteroids. Studies of the factors that regulate carbohydrate metabolism (termed glucocorticoids) culminated with the synthesis of cortisone, the first biologically active glucocorticoid to be available in large amounts. Subsequently, **Tate and colleagues** isolated and characterized a distinct corticosteroid aldosterone, that had potent effects on fluid and electrolyte balance (and therefore was termed mineralocorticoid).

The isolation of distinct corticosteroids that regulated carbohydrate metabolism or fluid and electrolyte balance ultimately led to the concept that the adrenal cortex comprises two largely independent units, an outer zone that produces mineralocorticoids and an inner region that synthesizes glucocorticoids and weak androgens.

Studies of the adrenal corticosteroids also played a key part in delineating the role of the anterior pituitary in endocrine function.

During the decades following **1930**, there was an intensive search for the active principles that could account for the essential role of the adrenal gland.

Reichstein and Von Euw (1937) prepared dexamethasone synthetically and demonstrated its presence in adrenal glands. Although this steroid had powerful effect on salt and water metabolism and became useful in the management of Addison's disease, it was obvious that extracts of adrenal cortex also contained compounds that in addition to affecting salt transport, could influence the metabolism of carbohydrates and proteins

World war II stimulated interest in the glucocorticoids, previously isolated by Kendall at the Mayoclinic. It was suspected that such compounds might be valuable in the treatment of shock and exhaustion. Intense efforts were made to synthesize amounts of glucocorticoids adequate for clinical trials.

Hench and Co-workers (1949) reported the effectiveness of cortisone and corticotropin in the treatment of rheumatoid arthritis. They observed that patients with rheumatoid arthritis tended to improve when patient was jaundiced or pregnant. They attributed this improvement to an antirheumatic factor of the adrenal gland. Results of the clinical trial, in rheumatoid arthritis were dramatic and soon cortisone and also corticotropin were found to cause symptomatic improvement in an amazing number of disease conditions. It was recognized at the same time that cortisone was not a cure for these many diseases. It seemed to provide the susceptible tissue with a shield like buffer against the irritant.

Subsequent research on the glucocorticoids led to the development of a variety of new steroids that have significantly greater antiinflammatory potency than cortisone, although their influence on carbohydrate metabolism generally parallels with antiinflammatory activity. A significant advance in newer steroids such as prednisone, methylprednisolone, triamcinolone and dexamethasone is that they exert little effect on renal sodium reabsorption, while possessing anti-inflammatory effect.

*

ANATOMY OF ADRENAL GLANDS

Suprarenal Glands (Adrenal gland)

The suprarenal glands or adrenal glands rest like cocked hats, on the superior surfaces of the kidneys[11]. These glands lie anterosuperior to the upper part of each kidney. They are somewhat asymmetrical, yellowish in colour weighing about 4gm, and lie within their own compartment of the renal fascia. Adrenal gland is an alternative name to the supra renal gland. The right supra renal gland is pyramidal in shape and surmounts the upper pole of the right kidney. It lies between the inferior venacava and the right crus of the diaphragm and encroaches on to the front of the right kidney. The anterior surface is in contact with the inferior venacava medially, above with the bare area of the liver and is covered below by the peritoneum of the posterior wall of the hepatorenal pouch.

The left supra renal gland is crescentric in shape and drapes over the medial border of the left kidney above the hilum. It lies on the left crus of the diaphragm adjacent to left inferior phrenic artery. The surface is covered by the peritoneum of the posterior wall of the lesser sac, forming part of the stomach bed. Its lower part is in contact with the body of the pancreas and the splenic vessels.

Blood supply :

Both the glands receive blood from 3 sources: from the aorta, from the renal and inferior phrenic arteries. In contrast, there is usually a single vein. The right vein is only a few millimeters long and enters the vena cava; the left vein is longer and enters the left renal vein. In each case the suprarenal vein drains into a persisting segment of the subcardinal vein of the embryo.

Lymphatic Drainage :

To para – aortic nodes.

Nerve supply :

The main supply is by myelinated preganglionic sympathetic fibers from the splanchnic nerves via the aortic and renal plexus; the fibers synapse directly with medullary cells. Blood vessels in all parts receive the usual postganglionic sympathetic supply, although cortical control is not neural but by ACTH from the anterior pituitary.

Structure :

Adrenal gland is composed of two distinct structural and functional components, the cortex and the medulla. The cortex develops from the mesoderm and the medulla from ectoderm. The outer part of the gland, the cortex, has a distinctly different appearance from the inner portion the medulla. The cortex, whose principal products are cortisol, aldosterone, androgens and related hormones, consists of three layers or zones. Immediately beneath the connective tissue capsule is the zona glomerulosa, with small rounded groups of cells. the second layer is the largest of the three, the zona fasciculata, consisting of parallel rows of pale-staining vacuolated cells with a high cholesterol content. The innermost is the zona reticularis, which is made up of a network of smaller and darker-staining cells. The rather small central medulla has larger cells secreting the catecholamines: adrenaline (80%) and noradrenaline (20%) and some dopamine. Many of the medullary cells exhibit the chromaffin reaction: they contain fine cytoplasmic granules (the catecholamine precursors) which are coloured brown by chromium salts. Dilated capillaries are usually prominent in the medulla but not in the cortex; as in any endocrine tissue, many capillaries are present but are collapsed in histological sections.

Embryology :

The adrenal gland develops from two distinct sources that produce separate organs in fish, but are combined in mammals. The medulla is derived from ectodermal cells, which migrate from the neural crest to their final location inside the adrenal cortex. The cortex is formed during the 4th – 6th week of fetal life from cells of coelomic mesoderm between the roots of the mesenteric and the genital ridge. Thus the adrenal cortex is derived from cells in close relation to those, which eventually form the ovary and testis. All these cells synthesize steroids, which may be precursors of hormones or actual hormones, which enter the circulation and produce the characteristic effect on ovaries, testicular or adrenocortical endocrine function. During fetal life the adrenal cortex is a relatively large organ (at 8 week it may be larger than the kidney) and the cells depend on ACTH stimulation, the cortisol secreted by the placenta. After birth, the adrenal cortex atrophies. The 3 different zones are not formed until 3 yrs of life.

*

HORMONES OF ADRENAL CORTEX

The adrenal cortex secretes a group of hormones called corticosteroids. Adrenal corticosteroids are necessary for regulation of homeostatic process. The adrenal cortex secretes and synthesizes more than thirty steroid hormones. Majority of these are classified into 2 groups on the basis of their actions as :

- ***Mineralocorticoids :*** Which affect the electrocytes of the extracellular fluid. Eg : Aldosterone – the principal compound.
- ***Glucocorticoids :*** are highly active compounds involved in the carbohydrate, protein, lipid and purine metabolism ; electrocyte balance and the functioning of most organs and tissues. They also possess anti– inflammatory and immune suppressive properties. Eg: Cortisol and corticosterone.

In addition to these, small amounts of sex hormones are secreted, especially androgenic hormones, which exhibit approximately, the same effects in the body as the male sex hormone testosterone.

Chemistry of Adrenocortical Secretion :-

All the adrenal cortical hormones are steroid compounds. The basic structure of a steroid is a complex cyclopentanophenanthrene ring with various functional groups attached to different carbon atoms. Most naturally occuring steroids contain alcohol side chains and are referred to as sterols.

All steroidal hormones have similar basic structure, with relatively minor differences, which however cause striking alterations in their biological activity.

They are sparingly soluble in water and, unlike most peptide hormones, circulate in association with binding proteins. They are soluble in lipids and in various organic solvents.

All the steroids can be synthesized basically from 2 – carbon acetate chains via cholesterol. The precursor for all adrenocortical hormones is cholesterol.

The adrenal cortex, derives its cholesterol requirement by uptake of low density lipoproteins from the circulation, which get bound to specific plasma membrane receptors and get transferred into the cells by the endocytosis. Cholesterol is largely esterified and stored in cytoplasmic vacuoles.

Cholesterol is also synthesized in adrenal cells from acetylcoenzyme A (acetylCoA) by usual pathway. Under basal circumstances, free cholesterol from plasma is the most direct and major source used for hormone synthesis.

All the steps that occur in the synthesis of steroid products take place in two organelles of the cell – the mitochondria and endoplasmic reticulum.

Each step is catalyzed by a specific enzyme system, and a change in even a single enzyme in the scheme can cause vastly different types of hormones to be formed.

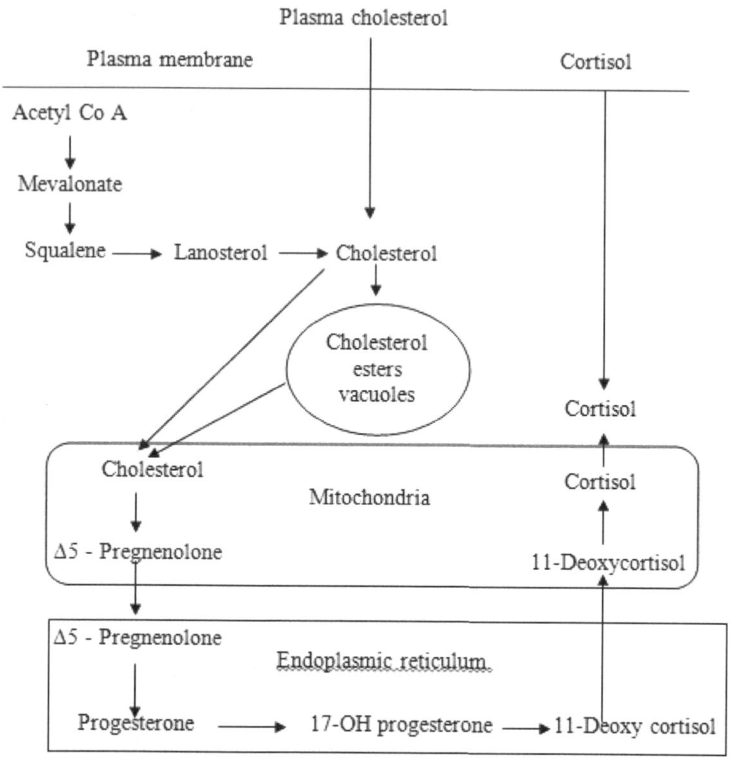

Intracellular reactions involved in the cortisol Biosynthesis

Glucocorticoids : The synthesis of glucocorticoids occurs largely in the zona fasciculata with a smaller contribution from zona reticularis.

Cortisol is the glucocorticoid for humans and most mammals, whereas corticosterone serves this function in some rodents. However, if cortisol synthesis is blocked, but the pathway to corticosterone is open, increased synthesis of the latter can provide the necessary glucocorticoid activity in humans.

The initial reaction converting cholesterol to Δ5 – pregnenolone is catalysed by a P-450 enzyme complex known as desmolase. This Δ5 – pregnenolone is then converted to 11-deoxycortisol by successive steps within the endoplasmic reticulum. The latter steroid is hydroxylated in the 11 position after transfer back to the mitochondria. The end product, cortisol, rapidly diffuses out of the organelle and then out of the cell. The last and critical step for glucocorticoid synthesis, 11-hydroxylation is very efficient in humans, 95% of the 11-deoxycortisol formed is converted to cortisol.

Mineralocorticoids : The synthesis and secretion of aldosterone, the major mineralocorticoid, is carried out exclusively by the zona glomerulosa. The transformation from cholesterol to corticosterone is identical to that in the zona fasciculata. The C_{18} methyl group of corticosterone is then oxidized by mitochondrial P-450 enzyme to yield aldosterone, which is rapidly released. The conversion of the 18 methyl group to an aldehyde is carried out by the same enzyme that is responsible for 11-hydroxylation in the zona fasciculata.

It is the oxygen atom bound at the number18 carbon of the cholesterol nucleus that is most important in providing the mineralocorticoid activity of aldosterone. The gluco-corticoid activity of cortisol is provided principally by the presence of keto-oxygen on carbon number 3 and the hydroxylation of carbon number 11 and 21.

Androgens and estrogens : The synthesis of sex steroids occurs largely in the zona reticularis, although zona fasciculata possesses the same capabilities. The 17 hydroxylated derivatives of Δ5-pregnenolone and progesterone are the starting points for androgen and estrogen synthesis. Removal of C_{20-21} scale chains is the key step yielding dehydroepiandrosterone (DHEA) and androstenedione. DHEA is then sulfated by a specific enzyme. Dehydroepiandrosterone sulfate (DHEA-S) and DHEA are the major androgenic products of the adrenal gland.

The major steps in the synthesis of the three principal adrenal steroids can be summarized as :

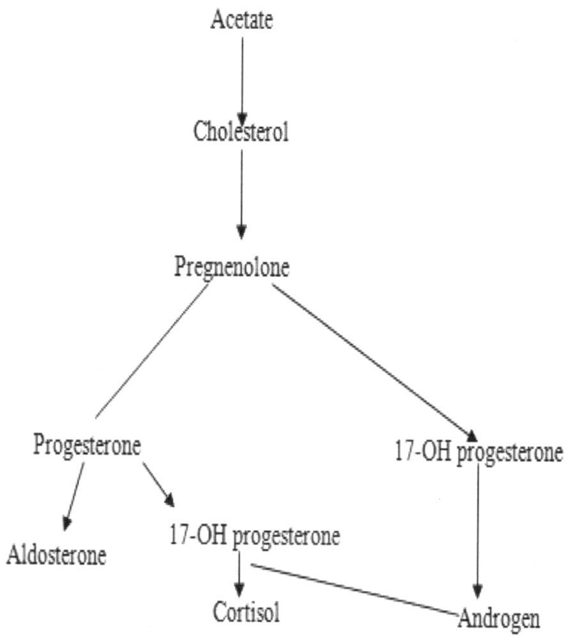

The important adrenal cortical hormones are :

Mineralocorticoids :

- Aldosterone (very potent, accounts for nearly 90% of mineralocorticoid activity)

- Desoxycorticosterone (one fifth as potent as aldosterone, very small quantities secreted)
- Corticosterone (slightly active)
- Cortisol (very slight activity but large quantities secreted)

Glucocorticoids :

- Cortisol (very potent, accounts for about 95% of all glucocorticoid activity)
- Corticosterone (about 4% of total glucocorticoid activity, but much less potent than cortisol).

*

REGULATION OF ACTH

ACTH AND REGULATION OF ACTH SECRETION

ACTH – the adrenocorticotropic hormone is one of the six very important hormones secreted by the anterior pituitary gland. The anterior pituitary gland contains many different types of secretory cells-like the somatotropes, corticotropes, thyrotropes, gonadotropes and lactotropes. The corticotropes secrete ACTH and they constitute about 20% of the cells of the anterior pituitary gland.

Chemistry of ACTH

ACTH is a straight chain polypeptide of molecular weight 45,000 containing 39 aminoacids. Only the first 23 aminoacids are required for their activity and remain same in all species. The remaining 16 aminoacids are biologically inactive.

Removal of a single aminoacid at the amino terminus considerably impairs biological activity. A number of aminoacids can be removed from the carboxy-terminal and without a marked effect. First 19 aminoacids are sufficient for stimulating hydrocortisone production.

ACTH is synthesized as a part of a larger precursor protein – pro-opiomelanocortin (POMC) and is liberated from the precursor by proteolysis. A number of other biologically important peptides, including endorphins, lipotropins and the melanocyte stimulating hormones (MSH), are also produced from the same precursors. The first 13 aminoacids in ACTH are the same as in melanocyte stimulating hormone, and so, ACTH can exert its effect on melanocytes.

Functions

1) It stimulates the synthesis of corticosteroids by the adrenal gland and also enhances their release from that gland.
2) It increases the total protein synthesis.
3) It causes the synthesis of steroid hormone from cholesterol.
4) It has a mild stimulating effect in dispersing melanin granules on the skin.
5) Administration of ACTH causes
    a) Increased excretion of nitrogen, potassium and phosphorous
    b) Retention of sodium, chloride and secondary retention of water
    c) Elevation of fasting blood sugar.
    d) Increase in circulating free fatty acids
    e) Increased excretion of uric acid
    f) Decline in circulating eosinophils and lymphocytes.
6) Since it activates adenylate cyclase and increases intracellular levels of cAMP, it can increase lypolysis in adipose tissue and stimulate insulin secretion from the pancreas.

7) Puromycin, the blocking agent of protein synthesis, inhibits the effect of ACTH on the adrenal gland.

Effect of ACTH on adrenal cortex

ACTH stimulates the adrenal cortex to secrete glucocorticoids, mineralocorticoids and weak androgens.

Functionally, the adrenal cortex comprises of two distinct compartments: the outer zona glomerulosa, which secretes the mineralocorticoid aldosterone, and the inner zona fasciculata / reticularis, which secretes glucocorticoid cortisol as well as adrenal androgens. The biological basis for these differences in steroidogenic output is that – the cells of the outer zone have receptors for angiotensin II and express aldosterone synthesis – an enzyme that catalyzes the terminal reactions in mineralocorticoid biosynthesis. In contrast, cells of the inner zone lack receptors for angiotensin II and express two enzymes steroid 17 α-hydroxylase ($P450_{17\alpha}$) and 11-β-hydroxylate ($P450_{11\beta}$) that catalyze the production of glucocorticoids.

In the absence of the adenohypophysis, the inner zone of the cortex atrophy, and the production of glucocorticoids and adrenal androgens are markedly impaired. Although ACTH acutely can stimulate synthesis of mineralocorticoid production by the zona glomerulosa, this zone is regulated predominantly by angiotensin II and extracellular K^+ and does not undergo atrophy in the absence of ongoing stimulation by the pituitary gland.

Persistently elevated levels of ACTH, due to either repeated administration of large amounts of ACTH or to excessive endogenous ACTH production induce hyperplasia and hypertrophy of the inner zones of the adrenal cortex with overproduction of cortisol and adrenal androgens.

Adrenal hyperplasia is most marked in congenital disorders of steroidogenesis, where ACTH levels are continuously elevated as a secondary response to impaired cortisol biosynthesis.

An important component of the tropical effect of ACTH is the enhancement of transcription of genes that encode the individual steroidogenic enzymes, with associated increase in the steroidogenic capacity of the gland.

Although the molecular mechanisms are still under investigation, it appears that a variety of different transcriptional regulators mediate the induction of the steroid hydroxylase by ACTH.

Regulation of ACTH secretion

Hormonal secretion by the adrenal cortex is controlled by the feedback system of the hypothalamus-pituitary-adrenal axis. Fluctuations in the rates of secretion of glucocorticoids are determined by fluctuations in the release of ACTH by the pituitary corticotropes. These corticotropes, in turn, are regulated by corticotropin releasing hormone (CRH). CRH is a peptide hormone formed by hypothalamus and reaches the anterior pituitary by the portal circulation.

CRH is secreted into the primary capillary plexus of the hypophyseal portal system in the median eminence of the hypothalamus and then carried to the anterior pituitary gland, where it induces ACTH secretion. The cell bodies of neurons that secrete CRF are located mainly in the paraventricular nucleus of the hypothalamus. This nucleus in turn receives many nervous connections from the limbic system and lower brain stem.

The anterior pituitary gland can secrete only minimum quantities of ACTH in the absence of CRF. Instead, most conditions that cause high ACTH secretory rates initiate this secretion by signals that begin in the basal regions of the brain, including the hypothalamus, and are then transmitted by CRF to the anterior pituitary gland.

The three organs – hypothalamus, anterior pituitary and adrenal cortex are together known as the hypothalamo-pituitary-adrenal axis (HPA), an integrated system that maintains appropriate levels of glucocorticoids.

There are three characteristic levels of regulation of the HPA axis:

- The diurnal rhythm is basal steroidogenesis
- Negative feedback regulation by adrenal corticosteroids
- Marked increase in steroidogenesis in response to stress.
- Initially increase and then return to normal – a phenomenon termed ACTH escape.

Mechanism of action :

ACTH stimulates the synthesis and release of adrenocortical hormone. As specific mechanisms for steroid hormone secretion have not been defined and since steroids do not accumulate appreciably in the gland, it is believed that the action of ACTH to increase steroid hormone production are predominantly mediated at the level of de novo biosynthesis.

ACTH initiates its action by binding to an adrenal plasma membrane receptor, a member of the G-protein receptor family, closely resembling in its structure are the receptors for melanocyte stimulating hormone. ACTH acts through the G protein GS to activate adenyl cyclase in a Ca^{++} - dependent manner and increase intracellular cAMP content. The concentration of cAMP in the cells reaches a maximum in about 3 minutes.

There is evidence suggesting that one subsequent event in the phosphorylation of ribosomal protein or proteins, the latter in turn, may control the translation from messenger RNA of another labile regulatory protein capable of activating a key cytochrome P-450 enzyme.

ACTH also increases adrenal phosphatidyl inositol turnover, and this second messenger system may participate in mediating the stimulation of steroid synthesis.

The most important action of ACTH is to stimulate the rate limiting desmolase reaction, which causes initial conversion of cholesterol to pregnenolone.

This explains why ACTH normally is necessary for any adrenocortical hormone to be formed.

The adrenal cortex uses multiple sources of cholesterol to ensure an adequate supply of substrate for steroidogenesis. These sources include

1) Circulating cholesterol and cholesterol esters taken up via the CDL receptor pathway.

2) Liberation of cholesterol from endogenous cholesterol ester stores via activation of cholesterol esterase.

3) Increased denovo biosynthesis.

The mechanism by which ACTH causes - the circadian rhythm (CR) is not known although some discrete data are available. Thus, CR is related to the sleep- wake cycle as well as light and darkness cycle. CR is not established in infants (who sleep often in the day and keep long spells of waking in the night) or in the blind.

The neurotransmitter, dopamine might be involved in the causation of CR. Thus, depletion of dopamine in the hypothalamus by the drug cytoheptadine abolishes CR. CR is also related to the time of food intake.

Diurnal Rhythm / Circadian Rhythm :

Plasma ACTH levels undergo diurnal fluctuations resulting in fluctuations in the adrenocortical activity. The diurnal rhythm is entrained by higher neuronal centers in response to sleep-wake cycles, such that levels of ACTH peak in the early morning hours, causing the circulating glucocorticoid levels to peak at approximately 6-8 a.m, declines during the day and reaches a minimum at about midnight. The plasma cortisol level ranges between a high of about 20μg / dl an hour before arising in the morning and a low of about 5 μg/dl around the midnight. When a person changes daily sleeping habits, the cycle changes correspondingly.

Negative feedback of glucocorticoids :

Glucocorticoids inhibit ACTH secretion via direct and indirect actions on CRH neurons to decrease CRH mRNA levels and CRH release and via direct effects on corticotropes. The effect on CRH release may be mediated by specific corticosteroid receptors in the hippocampus, which are proposed to play important roles in negative feed back inhibition exerted by glucocorticoids. At lower cortisol levels, the mineralocorticoid (type I) receptor, which have a high affinity for glucocorticoids and is primarily localized to the hippocampus, is the major species occupied. As glucocorticoid concentrations rise, the glucocorticoid (type II) receptors also become occupied as the capacity of the mineralocorticoid receptor is exceeded. Basal activity of the HPA axis apparently is controlled by both classes of receptor, whereas feedback inhibition by glucocorticoids predominantly involves the glucocorticoid receptor.

In the pituitary, glucocorticoids act through the glucocorticoid receptor to inhibit the expression of POMC (pro-opiomelanocortin) in corticotropes, as well as the release of ACTH. These effects are both rapid (occurring within seconds to minutes and possibly mediated by glucocorticoid receptor – independent mechanism) and delayed (requiring hours and involving changes in gene transcription mediated through the glucocorticoid receptor).

The stress Response :

Circumstances of stress overcome negative feedback regulation of the HPA axis, leading to a marked rise in the production of corticosteroids. Any type of physical or even mental stress can lead within minutes to greatly enhanced secretion of ACTH and consequently of cortisol as well, often increasing cortisol secretion as much as 20 fold.

Examples of stress signals include injury, hemorrhage, severe infection, major surgery, hypoglycemia, cold, pain and fever. The output during medical stress approaches 60 mg. Although precise mechanism that underlie this stress response and the essential actions played by the glucocorticoids are not defined fully, it is clear that glucocorticoid secretion is vital for maintaining homeostasis in these stressful settings.

It is believed that pain stimuli caused by the stress are first transmitted upward through the brain stem to the perifornical area of the hypothalamus and from here into area of the hypothalamus and eventually to the median eminence, where CRF is secreted into the hypophyseal portal system. Within minutes the entire control sequence leads to large quantities of glucocorticoids in the blood.

Mental stress can also cause equally a rapid increase in ACTH secretion. This is believed to result from increased activity in the limbic system, especially in the region of the amygdala and hippocampus, both of these then transmitting signals to the posterior medial hypothalamus.

Stress can override the circadian rhythm as well as negative mechanism. If the stress is extremely severe, the plasma cortisol level falls and this usually heralds death.

In nut shell, regulation of ACTH release is determined largely by the influence of blood hydrocortisone. Concentration on CRF production through negative feedback - Stressful stimuli, including drugs such as epinephrine, can override the feedback inhibition, release CRF and ACTH, and elevate the hydrocortisone concentration. In addition to these important regulatory influences, there is a diurnal variation in ACTH release.

*

METABOLISM AND EXCRETION OF ADRENAL CORTICOIDS

The adrenal corticoids circulate in the plasma partly free and mostly bound to proteins. The free form is biologically active and the bound portion is a reserve form. Cortisol circulates in plasma 75% to 80% bound to a specific corticosteroid binding L_2 globulin called transcortin. This glycoprotein has a molecular weight of 52,000 and binds a single molecule of cortisol. The normal concentration of transcortin is 3mg/dl, with a binding capacity of 20 μg cortisol/dl. An additional 15% of plasma cortisol is bound to albumin, leaving only 5-10% free.

The concentration of transcortin is increased during pregnancy and by estrogen administration; thus total plasma cortisol is increased in these conditions. The plasma half life of cortisol is about 70 min, and the metabolic clearance rate averages 200 L/day. The free fraction of cortisol in plasma is filtered by the kidney, but only about 0.3% of the total daily secretion, or approximately 50 μg is excreted in the urine in this manner.

The combined and the free forms of the hormones are transported through the extracellular compartment. Cortisol is in equilibrium with its 11-keto analogue cortisone. This interconversion is catalyzed by11β-oldehydrogenase which is present in many tissues. The glucocorticoid activity of cortisone is dependent on its conversion to cortisol. The vast majority of cortisol and cortisone is metabolized in the liver; the metabolites then are conjugated and excreted in the urine as glucuronides. The corticosteroids being water insoluble are excreted in urine only in traces.

The measurement of urinary metabolites provides a reliable index of cortisol secretion as long as hepatic and renal functions are intact.17-hydrocorticoids comprises upto 50% of the total daily cortisol secretion. The normal value ranges from 2-12 mg/day. The values are slightly higher in men than in women, as are cortisol secretion rates. Measurement of urinary 17-hydroxycorticoids (or urinary free cortisol) is used to assess adrenocortical responsiveness to ACTH stimulation or its suppressibility to exogenous synthetic glucocorticoids.

The cortisol precursors, progesterone and 17-hydroxy progesterone, are metabolized to cortisol analogus to those of cortisol. The excretory products are known as pregnanediol and pregnanetriol, respectively.

In adult females, measurement of these urinary metabolites reflects both adrenal and ovarian secretion. In pre pubertal children, however, elevation of urinary pregnanetriol specifically indicates increased secretion of adrenal17-hydroxyprogesterone and is, therefore, a valuable marker for congenital blocks in cortisol secretion.

Aldosterone circulates in plasma bound to a specific aldosterone binding globulin, to transcortin and to albumin. Overall binding is weaker than for cortisol.[79,42] Hence, the plasma half life is only 20 minutes, and the metabolic clearance rate is 1,600 L/day. 90%of the aldosterone is cleared by the liver in a single passage.

In the liver, aldosterone is reduced to tetrahydroaldosterone, the major metabolite that is excreted in the urine as the 3-glucuronide. A small portion of aldosterone is simply excreted as the 18-glucuronide. 18-glucuronide, is the urinary form that is commonly measured. The values in subjects with a normal sodium diet range from 5-20μg/day.

Androsterone, etiocholanolone and DHEA-S together makeup the major part of a urinary fraction called 17-ketosteroids. Normal values range from 5-14 mg/day in women to 8-20 mg/day in men A large increase in urinary 17-ketosteroid excretion almost always indicates an adrenal abnormality.

*

GLUCOCORTICOSTEROIDS

Physiological functions and pharmacological effects :

The effects of corticosteroids are numerous and wide spread. Their diverse effects include :

- Alteration in carbohydrate, protein and lipid metabolism.
- Maintenance of fluid and electrocyte balance
- Preservation of normal function of the cardiovascular system, the kidney, skeletal muscle, hematopoesis, endocrine system and nervous system.

In addition, by the mechanisms that are still not fully understood, corticosteroids endow the organism the capacity to resist stressful circumstances such as noxious stimuli and environmental changes.

The net effect of its metabolic actions is catabolic or antianabolic.

Until recently, corticosteroid effects were viewed as physiological – reflecting actions of corticosteroids at doses corresponding to normal daily production levels (or)

Pharmacological representing effects seen only at doses exceeding the normal daily production of corticosteroids.

More recent concept suggests that the anti-inflammatory and immunosuppressive actions of corticosteroids – One of the major pharmacological use of this class of drugs provide a protective mechanism in the physiological settings. Since many of the immune mediators associated with the inflammatory response decrease vascular tone and could lead to cardiovascular collapse if unopposed by the adrenal corticosteroids.

This hypothesis is supported by the fact that the daily production rate of cortisol can rise markedly (at least 10 folds) in the setting of severe stress. In addition, the pharmacological actions of corticosteroids or in different tissues and many of their physiological effects seem to be mediated by the same receptors.

Thus, the various glucocorticoid derivatives used as pharmacological agents have side effects on physiological processes that parallel their therapeutic effectiveness.

The actions of corticosteroids are related in a complex way to those of other hormones. The term 'permissive' has been used to describe many actions of cortisol, implying that the hormone may not directly initiated so as they allow certain processes to occur.

This concept may help to explain the need for the hormones critical yet unfocussed presence. Some of the examples that can better define this permissive role are :

1) Cortisol may amplify the effect of another hormone in a process that it does not by itself stimulate glycogenolysis. However, cortisol augments the stimulation of glycogenolysis by glucagons.

2) Cortisol and glucagons individually increase the activity of enzyme phosphoenolpyruvate, carboxylkinase. However, their combined effect is

more than additive i.e, cortisol synergizes with glucagons in their important step of gluconeogenesis.

General mechanism for corticosteroid effects :

Corticosteroids interact with specific receptor proteins in target tissues to regulate the expression of corticosteroid – responsive genes, there by changing the levels and array of proteins synthesized by various target tissues. As a consequence of the term required for changes in gene expression and protein synthesis, most effects of corticosteroids are not immediate, but become apparent after several hours. This fact is of clinical significance because a delay generally is seen before any beneficial effects of corticosteroids become manifested.

Corticosteroids predominantly act to increase the expression of target genes. However, there are well documented examples where glucocorticoids decrease transcription of target genes. In contrast to these genetic effects recent studies have raised the possibility that some actions of corticosteroids are immediate and are mediated by membrane bound receptors.

Glucocorticoid receptors :

Glucocorticoid receptors reside predominantly in the cytoplasm in an inactive form. Steroid binding results in receptor activation and translocation to the nucleus. The inactive glucocorticoid receptor is found as a complex with other proteins, including heat shock protein HSP 70 and a 56 – kDa immunophilin. HSP 90 through interaction with the steroid binding domain may facilitate folding of glucocorticoid receptor into an appropriate conformation that is believed essential for ligand binding.

Regulation of Gene expression by glucocorticoids :

Following ligand binding HSP 90 and several other of the associated proteins and the glucocorticoid receptor termed glucocorticoid responsive elements and provide specificity to the induction of gene transcription by glucocorticoids.

Genes whose expression is negatively regulated by glucocorticoids also have been identified. Genes that are negatively regulated by the glucocorticoids include those that code for a number of cytokines, regulatory molecules that play key role in the immune and inflammatory networks, and for collagenase and stromelysin, enzymes proposed to play key roles in the destruction of joints as seen in inflammatory arthritis.

Carbohydrate metabolism :

The best known metabolic effect of cortisol and other glucocorticoids on metabolism is their ability to stimulate gluconeogenesis (formation of carbohydrate from proteins and some other substances) by the liver often increasing the rate of gluconeogenesis as much as 6 – 10 folds. This results mainly from 2 different effects of cortisol.

1) All the enzymes required to convert amino acids into glucose are increased in the liver cells. This results from the effect of glucocorticoids to activate DNA transcription in the liver cell nuclei, that in

turn lead to an array of enzymes required for gluconeogenesis.

2) Cortisol causes mobilization of aminoacids from the extrahepatic tissues, mainly from the muscles. As a result, more amino acids become available in the plasma to enter into the gluconeogenesis process of the liver and there by promote the formation of glucose.

Decreased glucose utilization by cells :

Cortisol also causes a moderate decrease in the rate of glucose utilization by the cells everywhere in the body. The mechanism by which glucocorticoids inhibit glucose utilization in peripheral tissues are not fully understood. Glucocorticoids decrease glucose uptake in adipose tissue, skin, fibroblasts, thrombocytes and polymorphonuclear leukocytes.

These effects are postulated to result from the translocation of glucose transporters from the plasma membrane to an intracellular location. These peripheral effects are associated with a number of catabolic actions, including atrophy of lymphoid tissue, decreased muscle mass, negative nitrogen balance and thinning of skin.

Elevation of blood glucose concentration and adrenal diabetes :

Both the increased rate of gluconeogenesis and the moderate reduction in the rate of glucose utilization by the cells cause the blood glucose concentration to raise. The increase in concentration is occasionally great enough –

about 50% or more above normal – the condition is called "Adrenal diabetes".

Administration of insulin lowers the blood glucose concentration only to a moderate amount in adrenal diabetes not nearly, so much as it does in pancreatic diabetes. On the other hand, insulin causes greater decrease in blood glucose concentration in adrenal diabetes than in pituitary diabetes therefore, pituitary diabetes is said to be weakly insulin sensitive, adrenal diabetes moderately insulin sensitive and pancreatic diabetes strongly insulin sensitive. Therefore, cortisol is contraindicated in diabetics.

Effect on glycogen :

Cortisol plays a role in the defense against hypoglycemia. The rapid release of glycogenolytic hormones, glucagons and epinephrine is primarily responsible for the rapid recovery of plasma glucose levels. However, the prior action of cortisol leads to the build up of sufficient glycogen stores on which the other hormones can act.

In addition, cortisol amplifies both the glycogenolytic and gluconeogenic actions of glucagon and epinephrine. Also cortisol enhances glucagon release by the alpha cells of pancreatic islets.

Effects of cortisol on protein metabolism :

1) Reduction of cellular protein :

One of the principal effects of cortisol on the metabolic system of the body is reduction of the protein stores in essentially all body cells except those of liver. This is caused by both decreased protein synthesis and increased catabolism of proteins already present in the cells.

2) Increased liver protein and plasma protein :

Cortisol increases the blood production rates of both the essential aminoacid, lucine and the non-essential aminoacid, alanine, indicating protein breakdown. The increased production rates raise the plasma concentration of the branched chain aminoacid. Lower alanine levels do not rise because the conversion of alanine to glucose is almost markedly increased by cortisol.

Coincidentally with the reduced proteins elsewhere in the body the liver proteins become enhanced. Furthermore, the plasma proteins (which are produced by the liver and released into the blood) are also increased. Therefore, these are exceptions to the protein depletion that occurs elsewhere in the body. It is believed that this difference results from a possible effect of cortisol in enhancing amino acid transport into the liver producing enzymes required for protein synthesis.

Although the combined catabolic and antianabolic action of cortisol in normal amounts is physiologically beneficial, an excess of endogenous cortisol or any exogenous glucocorticoid produces a continuous drain on body protein stores most notably in muscle, bone, connective tissue and skin. This drain cannot be compensated by dietary protein because of the inhibition of protein synthesis.

In the presence of great excess of cortisol the muscles can become so weak that the person cannot rise from the squatting position. Finally the immunity functions of the lymphoid tissue can be decreased to a small fraction of normal.

Cortisol further stimulates the transformation of the proteolytically derived aminoacids into glucose precursors.

Glucocortioids are critical, to the survival of a fasting animal or human. Without them there is no increase in proteolysis during fasting as evidenced by lack of increase in urinary nitrogen excretion. Therefore when liver glycogen stores are depleted, gluconeogenesis from protein is deficient and death from hypoglycemia may ensue.

Cortisol decreases the formation of RNA in many extrahepatic tissues, especially muscles.

3) Increased blood amino acids diminished transport of amino acids into extrahepatic cells and enhanced transport into hepatic cells.

The decreased transport of aminoacids into extrahepatic cells decreases their intracellular aminoacid concentrations and as a consequence decreases the synthesis of protein. However, catabolism of proteins in the cells continues to release aminoacids from the already existing proteins and these diffuse out of the cell to increase the plasma aminoacid concentration. Therefore, cortisol mobilizes aminoacids from the nonhepatic tissues and diminishes the tissue stores of protein.

The increased plasma concentration of aminoacids, plus the cortisol enhanced transport of aminoacids into the hepatic cells, could also account for enhanced utilization of aminoacids by the liver to cause effects like

1) Increased rate of deamination of aminoacids by the liver.
2) Increased protein synthesis in the liver.
3) Increased protein synthesis formation of plasma proteins by the liver
4) Increased conversion of amino acids to glucose – that is enhanced gluconeogenesis.

Thus, it is possible that many of the effects of cortisol on the metabolic systems of the body result mainly from this ability of cortisol to mobilize aminoacids from the peripheral tissues while at the same time increasing the liver enzymes required for the hepatic effects by causing the formation of appropriate messenger RNAs.

Effects of cortisol on fat metabolism : Mobilization of fatty acids :

Cortisol promotes the mobilization of fatty acids from adipose tissue. This increases the concentration of free fatty acids in the plasma, which also increases the utilization for energy. Cortisol moderately enhances the oxidation of fatty acids perhaps results secondarily from the reduced availability of glycolytic products for metabolism. The mechanism by which cortisol promotes fatty acid mobilization is not yet understood. However, part of the effect probably results from diminished transport of glucose into the fat cells.

α-glycerophosphate, which is a derivative of glucose is required for both deposition and maintenance of triglycerides in the cells and in its absence of fat cells begin to release fatty acids.

The increased mobilization of fats by cortisol, combined with increased oxidation of fatty acids in the cells, helps shift the metabolic system of the cell in terms of starvation or other stresses from utilization of glucose for energy to utilization of fatty acids instead.

Ketogenic effect of cortisol :

Cortisol has a ketogenic effect. Ketosis doesn't develop because of cortisol except in conditions, such as when insulin is also deficient.

Obesity caused by cortisol :

Despite the fact that cortisol can cause a moderate degree of fatty acid mobilization from adipose tissue, excess of cortisol secretion frequently develops peculiar type of obesity, with excess deposition of fat in the chest and head regions of the body with loss from extremities giving a "buffalo-hump" for some and a round face – "a moon face".

It has been postulated that this obesity is due to the fact that cortisol intake and caloric intake and stimulates lipogenesis in some tissues of the body at a rate even more rapidly than it is mobilized and oxidized.

Effect on fluid and electrolyte balance :

Glucocorticoids also exert effects on fluid and electrolyte balance, largely due to permissive effects on tubular function and actions that maintain glomerular filtration rate. Glucocorticoids play a permissive role in the renal excretion of free water. In addition, glucocorticoids also exert multiple effects on calcium metabolism. In the gut, steroids interfere with calcium uptake by undefined mechanisms, while there is an increase in calcium excretion at the level of the kidney. These effects collectively lead to decreased total body calcium stores.

Hydrocortisone has a feeble salt retaining and potassium wasting effect. However, when large doses (300 mg\ 24 hrs) are used, sufficient salt retention occurs to make the concurrent use of a mineralocorticoid unnecessary.

Under certain circumstances, the newer synthetic steroids, dexamethasone, Betamethasone and Triamcinolone, may actually produce a marked sodium loss in the urine.

Cortisol is essential for excreting a water load. Inability to excrete water load can develop leading to water intoxication. This defect can be corrected by administration of a glucocorticoid.

Cardiovascular system :

A major action of corticosteroids on the cardiovascular system is to enhance vascular reactivity to other vasoactive substances.[80] Cortisol is required for the maintenance of blood pressure. Besides sustaining myocardial performance, the hormone permits normal responsiveness of arterioles to the constrictive action of catecholamines. Cortisol also helps to maintain blood volume by decreasing the permeability of the vascular endothelium and by a weak mineralocorticoid action that enhances sodium conservation.

The absence of glucocorticoids lead to increase in capillary permeability, inadequate vasomotor responses of smaller blood vessels and reduction in the cardiac output. Glucocorticoids not only potentiate the precursor response of blood vessels to adrenaline and noradrenaline but also protect the blood vessels from the toxic effect of the latter. In pharmacological doses, they have a positive iontropic action on the heart.

Hypertension is sometimes seen during chronic administration of glucocorticoids and in the patients with Cushings Syndrome in the latter condition, it is an important cause of death.

In Cushings syndrome there is hypertension where as in Addison's disease, there is hypotension. In total absence of adrenocorticosteroids adrenaline and noradrenaline fail to produce the vasospasm satisfactorily. Adrenocorticosteroids particularly cortisol helps adrenaline and noradrenaline to produce vasospasm. Also cortisol induced decreased capillary permeability is also a contributing factor. In CVS shock, therefore, analogues of cortisols are frequently used by the clinicians.

Central nervous system :

Receptors of cortisol are present in the brain, especially in the limbic system. In an unknown manner, cortisol modulates perceptual and emotional functioning. Cortisol has an important effect on mood and behaviour. Auditory, olfactory and gustatory acuity are accentuated by cortisol deficiency; this suggest that the hormone normally has a damping effect that may be important in preventing sensory over load and disorganized response. However, an excess of cortisol interferes with normal sleep and can elevate the mood strongly or depress it. In addition, the threshold for seizure activity may be lowered.

In Addisons disease depression of mood and irritability are common. Mechanisms by which corticosteroids affect neural activity are unknown. Recent studies suggest that steroids produced locally in the brain (termed neurosteroids) may regulate neuronal excitability.

Skeletal muscles :

Corticosteroids are connected with the normal functioning of the muscles. Permissive concentrations of corticosteroids are required for the normal functioning of skeletal muscle. In patients with Addisons disease weakness and fatigue are frequent symptoms and are believed to reflect mostly an inadequacy of the circulatory system or due to hypotension. Glucocorticoid excess, over a prolonged period, either secondary to glucocorticoid therapy or endogenous hypercortism, tends to cause skeletal muscle wasting via unknown mechanism. This effect is termed “steroid myopathy”.

Digestive system :

It is usually believed that cortisol increases gastric HCl secretion and exacerbates an already existing peptic ulcer. However, all the authors do not agree with this. It is possible that cortisol damages the barrier mechanism in the stomach, which normally prevents peptic ulcer formation.

Bone :

Cortisol inhibits bone formation by several functions:

1) The synthesis of type I collagen, the fundamental component of bone matrix, is reduced by cortisol.

2) The rate of differentiation of osteoprogenitor cells to active osteoblasts is decreased.

3) Cortisol decreases the absorption of calcium from the intestinal tract by antagonizing the action of 1, 25 (OH) and possibly also by diminished the synthesis of this active Vit. D metabolite.

4) Excretion of calcium by the kidney is enhanced.

The net result is to reduce the availability of calcium for bone mineralization. Finally cortisol increases the rate of bone resorption. Thus one major consequence of cortisol excess is an overall reduction in bone mass resulting in osteoporosis. This is particularly noticeable in the vertebra. Chronic usage of cortisol for therapeutic purpose can lead to pathological fracture of the vertebra. The calcium drainage from the bone (by cortisol) is facilitated by the proteolytic action on the bone proteinaceous matrix by the cortisol.

Effects on blood cells :

Cortisol causes rise of RBC count and Hb%. This is perhaps due to the fact that the cortisol inhibits the phagocytosis of older RBC's. When excess cortisol is secreted by the adrenal glands, polycythemia results and conversely, when adrenal gland secrete no cortisol, anemia often results.

Corticosteroids also affect circulating white blood cells. ACTH or glucocorticoids cause an increase in the number of circulating neutrophils. This occurs as a result of increased release from the marrow, diminished rate of removal from the circulation and increased demargination from vascular walls.

Cortisol also causes lymphocytopenia, eosinopenia and monocytopenia. A single dose of hydrocortisone leads to a decline of these circulating cells within 4 – 6 hrs, which persists for 24 hrs and results from the periphery rather than from increased destruction. Indeed a finding of lymphocytopenia or eosinopenia is an important diagnostic criteria for the over production of cortisol by the adrenal gland. Likewise, administration of large doses of cortisol causes significant atrophy of all the lymphoid tissues throughout the body, which in turn decreases the output of both T cells and antibodies from the lymphoid tissue. As a result the level of immunity for all foreign invaders of the body is decreased. This can occasionally lead to fulminating infection and death from diseases that otherwise would not be lethal.

On the other hand, this ability of cortisol and other glucocorticoids to suppress immunity, makes these among the most useful of all drugs to revert immunologic rejection of transplanted hearts, kidneys and other tissues.

Anti-inflammatory and immunosuppressive effects :

When tissues are damaged by trauma, or infection with bacteria they become inflamed. In some conditions, the inflammation is more damaging than the trauma or disease itself. Irrespective of the type of injury or insult the inflammatory response is suppressed by glucocorticoids. This is the basis of most of their clinical uses. The action is non specific, as the cause of inflammatory reaction is not controlled by the corticosteroids. It covers all components and stages of inflammation. This includes reduction of increased capillary permeability, local exudation, cellular infiltration, phagocytic activity and late responses like capillary proliferation, collagen deposition, fibroblastic activity and ultimately scar formation. However, once a fibrous tissue is formed, it is not dissolved by corticosteroids.

Although the use of glucocorticoids as inflammatory agents does not address the underlying cause of the disease, the suppression of inflammation is of enormous clinical utility and has made these drugs among the most frequently prescribed agents. Similarly glucocorticoids are of immense value in treating diseases that result from undesirable immunological reactions. These diseases range from conditions that predominantly result from hormonal immunity, such as transplantation rejection. The immunosuppressive and anti-inflammatory actions of glucocorticoids are inextricably linked, perhaps because they both largely result from inhibition of specific functions of leukocytes.

Multiple mechanisms are involved in the suppression of inflammation by glucocorticoids. When large amounts of cortisol are secreted or injected into a person, the cortisol has 2 basic anti-inflammatory effects :

1) It blocks the early stages of inflammatory process.
2) If inflammation has already begun, it causes rapid resolution of the inflammation and increased rapidity of healing.

Prevention of the development of inflammation :

Cortisol has a very special and important influence on the set of reactions evoked by tissue trauma, chemical irritants, foreign proteins and infection. The immediate local reaction consists of dilation of capillaries and changes in the endothelial cell membranes that enhance the trapping of circulating leukocytes at the site of injury. These reactions, mediated by prostaglandins, thromboxane and leukotrienes are profoundly inhibited by all glucocorticoids through depression of these mediators. This results because, cortisol decreases the activity of the enzyme phospholipase A_2, which releases arachidonic acid from its linkage to phosphatidyl choline. Arachidonic acid is the immediate precursor to prostaglandins, thromboxanes and leukotrienes and its production is the rate limiting step in the synthesis of these mediators of inflammation.

In addition, glucocorticoids stabilize lysosomal membranes, that is, cortisol makes it much more difficult than is normal for the membrane of the intracellular lysosomes to rupture. Therefore, most of the proteolytic enzymes that are usually released by damaged cells to cause inflammation, which are mainly stored in the lysosomes are released in greatly decreased quantity.

Corticosteroids decrease the permeability of the capillaries, probably as a secondary effect of the reduced release of proteolytic enzymes. This prevents loss of plasma into the tissues.

Cortisol decreases both migration of white blood cells into the inflamed area and phagocytosis of the damaged cells. These effects probably result from the fact that cortisol diminishes release of lysosomal enzymes and other substances from the damaged cells because of its ability to stabilize both the cell and lysosome membrane and inhibit the recruitment of the neutrophils and macrophages into the affected area. Glucocorticoids inhibit the production of plasminogen activator by neutrophils (this enzyme converts plasminogen to plasmin). Plasmin is thought to facilitate the entry of neutrophils into the area of inflammation by hydrolysis of fibrin.

Effect on allergy :

Cortisol blocks the inflammatory response in allergic reactions in exactly the same way that it blocks other types of inflammatory responses. The basic allergic reaction between antigen and antibody is not affected by cortisol and even some of the secondary effects of the allergic reaction still occur.

The corticosteroids do not seem to inhibit the phagocytosis of antigen by the macrophages but they interfere with its subsequent intracellular digestion.

Only enormous doses (150 – 200 mg of prednisolone per day) of such steroids alter gamma globulin production by the plasma cells in circulation.

As a part of the inflammatory response, the previously sensitized lymphocytes on meeting the sensitizing agent, produce soluble factors called lymphokines, Glucocorticoids suppress the production of IL – 1 by the monocytes and IL – 2 by the lymphocytes. It also suppresses the production of other lymphokines such as tumour necrotic factor.

Cortisol suppresses fever mainly because of its suppressive effect on IL – 1 which is one of the principal expectant to the hypothalamic temperature control system. The decrease temperature in turn reduces the degree of vasodilation.

Effect of cortisol in causing resolution of inflammation :

Even after inflammation has become well established, administration of cortisol can often reduce inflammation within hours to a few days. The immediate effect is to block most of the factors that are promoting the inflammation. Then the rate of healing is also enhanced. This probably results from those same, mainly undefined factors that allow the body to resist tissue damage, although corticosteroids do not in moderate doses interfere with antibody production nor with antigen antibody union or with liberation of histamine from the tissues damaged by such union. They suppress the inflammatory response to it. This action is important in the suppression of such allergic phenomena as urticaria, allergic rhinitis and allergic bronchial asthma.

Antistress action :

Stress develops when the person develops acute pain or severe infection, fever or receives injuries or develops acute anxieties. These are all noxious stimuli.

Stress causes destabilization of heomostasis. The danger of stress is that, if not controlled, by causing derangement of heomeostatic mechanisms it may lead to death.

Any type of physical or even mental stress can lead within minutes to greatly enhanced secretion of ACTH and consequently of cortisol as well, often increasing cortisol concentration as much as 20 fold. It appears that an elevated cortisol level is needed to battle with the stress. However, the exact interrelationship between stress and cortisol is not clear. Although, cortisol and ACTH are the most important ones, many other hormones (CRH, ADH, adrenaline) play important roles in stress. However, a very high rise of cortisol secretion can cause harm eg : Stress ulcers in the stomach, in experimental animals.

It is believed that pain stimuli caused by the stress are first transmitted upward through the brain stem to the perifornical area of the hypothalamus and from there into the paraventricular nucleus of the hypothalamus and eventually to the median eminence where CRF is secreted into the hypophyseal portal system.

Within minutes the entire cortisol sequence leads to large quantities of glucocorticoids in the blood.

Mental stress can also cause equally a rapid increase in ACTH secretion. This is believed to result from increased activity in the limbic system, especially in the region of the amygdala and hippocampus, both of these seen transmitting signals to the posterior medial hypothalamus.

Although exact mechanism of the protective action of cortisol in stress is not known one theory states that, because cortisol can inhibit the arachidonic acid metabolism (AAM) including prostaglandin production and thus inhibits the capillary permeability, the exodus from the blood to the tissue is prevented during stress. That is, cortisol prevents fluid loss from the vascular compartment and fall of blood volume.

Also, precursor of the ACTH molecule in the anterior pituitary is POMC, from which both ACTH and β endorphin molecules are released. β endorphin, blunts the perception of pain, and in addition it inhibits the cortisol secretion. Thus, there is an autoregulatory (-ve feedback) mechanism which ensures that no threatening amount of excess cortisol is secreted even during stress.

The most important side effect that occurs during prolonged administration of glucocorticols is adrenal atrophy and loss of normal function in the adrenal cortex. Exogenous glucocorticosteroids in circulation provide negative feedback, which inhibits the production of CRF and subsequent release of ACTH. With reduced or no hormonal secretion, the adrenal cortex has decreased output and loses its ability to respond to demand.

The degree of adrenal atrophy is dependent upon the dose of glucocorticoid, the route of administration, the duration of therapy, and the frequency of administration. Relatively small doses (less than 30mg. cortisone or the equivalent of another glucocorticoid) given daily for periods of less than 1 week have been shown to cause little alteration in pituitary-adrenal function. It is important to realize that different glucocorticoids exhibit different activity and thus have varying equivalent dosages.

During periods of stress the patient's requirement for glucocorticoids is increased and may exceed the fixed dose that the patient is taking. Since the patient's pituitary-adrenal system is unable to respond to this need, the patient is left in a state of acute adrenal insufficiency or "adrenal crisis".

Glick M (1989) stated that adrenal suppression by low-dose corticosteroids (LDC, considered to be under the physiologic limit of 24 to 30 mg/day) is debatable when treatment is given for less than 1 month. To date, no studies have adequately tested the adrenal response in patients given such a low short-term dosage.

Cases in which LDC are given for longer than 1 month have been the subject of numerous studies. Generally these studies point to an absence of adrenal suppression in patients given LDC for extended periods of time. In one study the HPA function was only tested 5 months after cessation of therapy, and it was determined to be normal. Morris and Jorgensen suggested that any amount of glucocorticosteroids causes at least partial adrenal suppression. However, to the authors, only one study had shown concrete data that point to adrenal suppression after LDC.

Contrary to prevailing belief, even with short-term, high-dose corticosteroids (HDC), adrenal suppression is transitory. In one study, 300mg / day of hydrocortisone was given to 11 healthy male subjects for 30 days. No HPA function depression was noticed 30 days after the corticosteroid administration was stopped. Most studies also show a return within 14 days of the HPA functin to stress stimuli, with Webb and Clark showing a return of the normal pituitary and adrenal functions 4 days after cessation of a 3-week course of 160 mg/day of hydrocortisone equivalent.

With long-term HDC a natural pituitary adrenal recovery was delayed up to 12 months. However, the HPA function was never challenged during this period. One study involving children shows that the degree of HPA suppression is directly related to the dosage of corticosteroids. Change of plasma cortisol levels were found to follow any change in dosage by 2 weeks. Within 2 weeks after cessation of glucocorticosteroid therapy, cortisol response was indistinguishable from that found among control individuals who had not received corticosteroid therapy. Livanou and colleagues suggest that administration of HDC is associated with a slower recovery of plasma hydrocortisol levels than that produced by dosages of lesser amounts. Suppression of endogenous cortisol secretion occurs within minutes of administration of any corticosteroid with systemic action. Sparkes indicates that large quantities of topical corticosteroids can result in transient adrenal suppression. This claim has been sustained by numerous works showing adrenal suppression as a function of duration, potency or dosage, and method of application to the skin.

ADVERSE REACTIONS :

Stimulation with ACTH results in increased production of cortisol which causes almost the same unwanted effects as treatment with cortisol itself or a synthetic analogue.

Harter et al (1963) stated that it was not been possible to obtain a glucocorticoid with good anti-inflammatory action and no diabetogenic activity. Administration of all glucocorticoids results in a negative nitrogen balance. It has been stated that myopathy and muscle wasting are more commonly found when triamcinolone or dexamethasone are used. The severity of the unwanted effects depends in general on the dosage and duration of treatment. This can be prevented to some extent by giving the corticosteroid in one dose on alternating days.

Prolonged treatment results in suppression of adrenal activity and induces atrophy of the adrenal cortex. Adrenal insufficiency can be caused in these patients by omission of the level dose, reduction of the dose below the level needed for 'physiological' substitution, or during stress when the dose is not increased or the adrenal cortex is unable to produce supplemental endogenous cortisol, because of adrenal atrophy or inability to secrete ACTH.

The number of reports on adverse effects of treatment with ACTH and with glucocorticoids continues to increase. It remains difficult to make a comparison between continuous administration of ACTH and various steroid compounds as regards the incidence of adverse effects, since this depends not only on the type and dosage of steroid compound used, but also to some extent on the underlying disease and the age of the patient.

1) Allergic reactions :

Wolfromm and Herman (1967) reported that ACTH preparations of animal origin may give rise to allergic reactions. Hypersensitivity to ACTH has been observed not only in patients who had previously been treated with it but also in patients who had never received it for diagnostic or therapeutic purposes. Hypersensitivity to ACTH may cause only dizziness, nausea and vomitting, but in several instances shock with circulatory failure has been observed.

Rosselin et al (1966) used the antigenicity of porcine ACTH to develop a radio-immunoassay for human ACTH.

(Fleischer et al (1967); Landon et al (1967) stated that prolonged treatment with porcine ACTH causes formation of antibodies and loss of stimulatory effect on the human adrenals.

(Singer and Dobrowolski (1965) proposed that it is highly improbable that glucocorticoids give rise to allergic reactions. Neverthless one case of anaphylactic shock after intranasal administration of hydrocortisone acetate has been described.

Blood :

Blood dyscrasias due to treatment with ACTH or corticosteroids are extremely rare. Leukocytosis during treatment with prednisolone has been mentioned.

According to **Diamond (1966)** there is sufficient information about the effects of long-term high-dosage corticosteroid treatment in suppressing activity of normal bone marrow and producing fatty infiltration or replacement of the haematopoietic tissue to advise strongly against its use unless there is expectation of benefit is considerable. This implies that long-term corticosteroid therapy is contra-indicated in patients with acute thrombocytopenic purpura or aplastic anaemia in whom no objective amelioration of the blood dyscrasia can be observed within 2 or 3 weeks. Even in conditions where long-term corticosteroid therapy seems indicated, the dosage should be carefully regulated at the lowest therapeutic level. If possible it should then be given on alternate days or for only part of the week, and the bone marrow should be studied at relatively frequent intervals while the patient is under such treatment. Only in this way can the deleterious effects of long-term corticosteroid treatment and particularly its harmful action on the blood building system be avoided.

2) Skin (systemic administration of steroids) :

Rosselin et al (1966) stated that infections of the skin, bacterial, fungal as well as viral may occur during treatment with steroids, independent of the route of administrations. Hypertrichosis and acne frequently occur during therapy with steroids. Treatment with ACTH may result in hyper-pigmentation like that seen in Addison's disease

Shuster et al (1967) stated that Corticosteroid treatment reduces the skin collagen in patients with rheumatoid arthritis.

Knoppers (1966) reported two cases of purpura that had resulted from treatment of asthmatic bronchitis with triamcinolone and prednisone.

Lucena et al (1966) stated that that long-term treatment leads to a rearrangement of fat distribution: in particular the occurrence of moon-face and buffalo-hump.

The formation of a 'dewlap', a reversible episternal accumulation of fat has been reported in 3 patients.

3) Gastrointestinal tract :

Hadnagy et al (1965); Laumonier et al (1966), (1966); Kelley and Regan (1966); Goksen and Hardy (1967); Cooke and Grossman (1966); Sun and Hollander (1966) stated that the association between ulcer formation and corticosteroid therapy is well established.

A number of studies in animals have been published. The question whether steroid treatment induces ulceration de novo or reactivates subclinical ulcer is still unsettled. The question, whether ulcer formation is dose-dependent remains unsolved.

Cooke (1967) according to one report the risk is less with a lower dosage; according to another study there is no difference **(Rausch-Strooman, 1965)**. Many authors suspect a higher frequency in women than in men. Gastrointestinal complaints arise not only with oral therapy but also when steroids are given by other routes. The duration of treatment is also without influence on the risk of ulcer formation **(Popa and Munteanu, 1966)**. The risk seems to be higher in patients with advanced cancer and terminal illness **(Schell. 1966)**.

Hart and Boardman, (1965) reported that the combination of indomethacin with prednisolone seems to increase the risk.

Oriente et al (1965); Mortimer (1965); Baszynki et al (1965) also reported perforation of the duodenum during treatment with steroids.

Pancreas :

Sztaba and Stoba (1965); Schrier and Bulger (1965); Andersen (1966); Boros and Lajos, (1966) reported Pancreatitis developing both early and late during treatment with glucocorticoids.

Ulcerative colitis :

Goethals and Vandenbroucke (1966) stated that treatment with steroids is valuable but has found that the risk of toxic megacolon and/or a perforation of the colon is considerable.

4) Urinary tract :

Klima and Ort (1966) presented reports indicating lesions resembling diabetic nodular glomerular sclerosis, analogous to cortisone-induced renal lesions in rabbits, are produced in patients with nephrotic syndrome treated with cortisone. An increase in the number of cells in the urine was also described in patients on long-term treatment with cortisone for asthma. Administration of ACTH to a 10-year-old boy who had been treated with steroids for nephrotic syndrome for 6 years, was followed by anuria, renal cortical necrosis and death. Renal function was not severely impaired in the period immediately preceding his final illness.

5) Cardiovascular system :

Administration of glucocorticoids with mineralocorticoid activity may understandably lead to salt and water retention, oedema and hypertension. Long-term treatment with steroids may be accompanied by the occurrence of arteritis of the small vessels. It is not clear whether the arteritis is caused by the underlying disease or causally related to the treatment with steroids. Most of the available evidence points to the first possibility.

ECG change: Both ACTH and glucocorticoids can reverse the bradycardia due to complete or partial AV-block. Thrombosis and thrombophlebitis –

Florkiewicz and Klamut, (1966) reported thrombophlebitis of the major veins attributed to prednisone therapy in three cases.

Kornell (1966) reported a case where generalized scleroderma treatment with prednisolone coincided with an acceleration of involvement of the myocardium.

6) Respiratory system :

Local irritation of the pharynx and the upper airway by aerosols containing steroids has been mentioned before.

Apparently the redistribution of fat during treatment with steroids may also occur in the upper mediastinum. Interstitial cell pneumonia was observed after 40 days of cortisone therapy in a 14-month-old boy.

7) Central nervous system :

Mental disturbances: Usually administration of glucocorticoids causes euphoria. The intensity of the change in mood depends on the dosage administered, the sensitivity of the patient and the underlying personality. Full-blown psychosis has been described. The mental abnormality may be accompanied by fear, depression or stupor. Patients with chronic adrenal insufficiency are particularly sensitive, even to the normal substitution dosage. High doses of ACTH may also induce psychosis

Neurological phenomena : Latent epilepsy can be made manifest by administration of corticosteroids. Long-term treatment may result in papilloedema and increased intracranial pressure, particularly in children. The symptoms may simulate those of a brain tumour. Intra thecal administration of corticosteroids can cause elevation of cerebral spinal fluid protein and carries a real risk of arachnoiditis.

Rome HP and Braceland FJ (1952) described four grades of psychological response to steroid treatment, which they felt were prototypic of all clinical presentations.

Clinical classification of psychological response to steroids:-

Grade	Definition
1	Mild euphoria, lessened fatigue, improved sensation, increased sense of intellectual capacity
2	Heightened euphoria. Patients are effusive, expansive, volatile, hypomanic; exhibit flight of ideas,
3	Different responses reflecting the ego characteristics of the patient, such as anxiety, phobia, rumination, obsessional preoccupation, hypomania or depression
4	Grossly psychotic reactions with hallucinations, delusions, extreme variations in mood

Garner HH and Falk AM (1967) described case of a patient who was treated with 100mg prednisone per day for a severe case of pemphigus vulgaris and who became extremely psychotic after 14 days. The patient began to have hallucinations and delusions; he was treated with 150 mg chlorpromazine per day. Because of the severity of the underlying disease, it was necessary to continue use of the steroids. Garner and Falk also reviewed the literature on steroid-induced psychosis and described the usual case as one in which an acute anxiety state preceded the psychotic state. They also stated that patients predisposed to psychiatric illness are more likely to become psychotic with use of steroids.

Steroid-induced psychosis may occur with doses commonly used to treat many inflammatory reactions. The clinician should be alert for the signs and symptoms and be prepared to treat them. While the risk of steroid-induced psychosis is present with the steroid regimen most commonly used in oral surgery, this complication in conjunction with short-term steroid therapy is rare.

Silva RG, Tolstunov L (1994) presented a case report illustrating acute mental disturbances in a 45 years old patient who received high-dose parenteral steroids while undergoing a major maxillofacial surgical procedure. Preoperatively, for prophylaxis of postoperative edema, the patient received IV dexamethasone.

The total cumulative dose of dexamethasone was 60 mg. On postoperative days 2 and 3, the patient showed mild anxiety and agitation, which were interpreted as signs of pain and controlled with morphine. On postoperative day 4, the patient was anxious and developed transient visual and auditory hallucinations.

Psychiatric consultation led to a diagnosis of mild delirium, possibly caused by the prolonged surgery or the large amount of analgesics received. The patient was treated with haloperidol 1 mg intramuscularly every hour of sleep and as needed for confusion, and his routine medications were continued.

On postoperative day 9, the patient became hyperverbal and aggressive and was placed under close psychiatric observation. Later, the patient punched three large holes in the wall of his room, attempted to jump through the window, and required restraints.

The following morning the patient was briefly lucid and oriented and could not explain what had happened the previous night.

	Time administered	**Dose (mg)**
Immediate preoperative	9:00 AM	12
Intraoperative	4:00	12
Postoperative	12:00 AM	12
Postoperative day 1	9:00	12
Postoperative day 2	9:00	8
Postoperative day 3	9:00	4

While continuing to demonstrate episodes of an inappropriate and aggressive nature, the patient was transferred to a psychiatric-medical ward for closer observation and perphenaxine was increased to 16 mg orally 4 times a day. His transfer diagnosis was steroid-induced psychosis.

8) Eyes :

Infections : The topical application of corticosteroids to the eye may exacerbate an existing infection and cause perforations. Corneal ablations should never be treated with steroids topically. Infections can be masked until extensive damage has occurred. The contamination of steroids with a local anaesthetia in particular is hazardous. Re-epithelialization of corneal defects is slowed down by steroid treatment.

Moses (1965); Francois et al (1966) warned against treating herpetic keratitis with a local corticosteroid preparation.

Increased ocular pressure and glaucoma :

Crompton (1966) stated that a number of reviews and case reports discuss the rise in intraocular pressure that may lead to glaucoma and finally blindness. Topical as well as systemic treatment with steroids has this effect.

The steroid most frequently used in local treatment has been dexamethasone, but the complication has also been reported with hydrocortisone. The dosage of systemic corticoid therapy resulting in this complication is usually not excessive, for example 29 mg prednisone. The complication may occur after several years of treatment. The etiology is not apparent; the tendency for induction of ocular hypertension seems to be determined genetically.

According to one report 30% of the general population are heterozygous carriers of the glaucoma gene, 5% are homozygotes and will eventually have glaucoma even when not treated with steroids.

People not carrying the gene show a minimal rise in intraocular pressure when challenged with topical corticosteroids.

Families of known open-angle glaucoma patients should be warned of the risk of steroids and urged to have periodic examinations.

Cataract: Reports relating cataracts to long-term corticosteroid treatment continue to appear.

Spencer and Andelman (1965); Kahoutek and Havelka (1966) reported that cataracts have occurred in patients with rheumatoid arthritis after systemic treatment, in children with nephrotic syndrome treated for longer than one year **(Dikshit and Avasthi, 1965; Draver et al., 1966)**, and in one case of pemphigus treated with only 14 mg cortisone daily for two years **(Thalabard et al., 1966)**. The cataract may be unilateral **(Neuschuler, 1966)**. Local treatment of the eye has been described to give both glaucoma and subcapsular cataract **(Kornblueth et al., 1966)**.

Other changes in the eyes : Some physicians have used chemosis as a sensitive index of steroid overdosage. Blue transparent sclerae have been seen in patients treated for scleritis and in children with stunted growth following long-term therapy. Changes in refraction have been described.

9) **Skin (topical administration of steroids) :**

Coskey and Bryan (1967) have reported incidences of contact dermatitis after topical administration of methylprednisolone.

Topical administration of hydrocortisone and prednisolone resulted in contact dermatitis Several authors have studied the systemic effects of topically applied corticosteroids.

Atrophy of the skin may also occur after local application of steroids. Treatment of chronic leg ulcers with fluocinolone acetonide 0.025% combined with neomycin resulted in the development of necrosis.

10) **Endocrine glands :**

Systemic treatment with ACTH and glucocorticoids can cause severe symptoms of Cushing's syndrome. This can occur even when steroids are used topically.

Hyperglycaemia and diabetes : Steroid diabetes is often seen when ACTH or glucocorticoids are administere. In many but not all of these patients the family history shows a predisposition to diabetes mellitus. The glycosuria in steroid-treated patients may be due to hyperglycaemia, to a lowered renal threshold for glucose or to both. One report discusses the diabetogenic effect of steroid therapy in virus hepatitis and suggests that glycosuria appears in parallel with a serious impairment of liver function.

The frequency of steroid diabetes in man has varied with different authors according to dosage, age of the patient, and the steroid used. In well controlled diabetics the administration of steroid may appreciably increase the need for insulin. This is true for topical as well as for systemic administration.

Thyroid : Administration of ACTH or cortisone may suppress the uptake or radioactive iodine to some extent, probably by diminishing TSH secretion. However, both hyperthyroidism and hypothyroidism have been seen in patients treated with steroids.

Parathyroid : The antagonism between parathyroids and hypercorticism is well known. Latent hypoparathyroidism may be unmasked by administration of corticosteroids. The phosphate retention occurring in renal failure caused by adrenal insufficiency may also make hypoparathyroidism manifest.

Disturbance of growth : Retardation of growth is a common finding in children in long-term steroid treatment. The closure of the epiphysis may be delayed.

Frantz and rabkin (1964) showed experimentally that administration of corticosteroids suppresses secretion of growth hormone.

Biochemical changes : The sodium-retaining properties of aldosterone, cortisone and desoxy-corticosterone are greater than those of the newer steroid drugs. The severity of the potassium loss induced depends partly on the amount of sodium in the diet. With the synthetic preparations the excretion of potassium is less marked. Administration of glucocorticoids leads also to the mobilization of calcium and phosphorous.

Osteoporosis : Osteoporosis and its sequelae continue to be reported as the most severe adverse effects of treatment with glucocorticoids. It is most severe in patients with restricted physical activity, e.g. in rheumatoid arthritis. The osteoporosis is usually generalized and may be seen as a motley skull, fish vertebrae, spontaneous fractures with hyperostotic callus, protrusio acetabuli, aseptic necrosis of the head of femur and humerus and an atrophy of the Charcot type. Intra-articular administration of steroids may result in destruction of the joint in osteo-arthrotic arthritis. It has been suggested that the destruction of the joint is caused by its intensive use when the pain is relieved by local or systemic therapy. Systemic administration of corticosteroids may also accelerate pre-existing multiple joint disease. The same alterations can be found in natural Cushing's syndrome. In one series of 60 paticnts with rheumatoid arthritis necrosis of the femoral head was seen in 10% after oral treatment with steroids only.

Spontaneous fractures, especially of the vertebrae and of the ribs, have been reported during steroid therapy. In one instance a fracture of the os pubis and os ischii has been described. Generalized osteoporosis may cause loss of height and cause vague rheumatic complaints.

11) Infections :

Treatment with glucocorticoids carries an increased risk of infection. Of course this is not the case when physiological doses of cortisone are used in patients with adrenal insufficiency.

Tuberculosis : Aggravation of existing tuberculosis and reactivation of completely quiescent / quiet stages of the disease is well known. In one series of 60 patients reactivation was seen in 6 within 2 months, in 13 within a year and in the rest within 3 years. 21 of them became infectious, 5 got miliary tuberculosis, 3 tuberculous infections of the joints. In 5 instances tuberculosis was the cause of death. Steroid therapy in combination with tuberculostatic agents has been used in critically ill patients with pulmonary tuberculosis.

Bacterial infections - Bacterial infections including sepsis, osteomyelitis, activation of periodontal lesions, suppurative arthritis after local injections and after oral administration have been reported. Bacteremia after topical use of prednisolone in infected pulps of monkeys has been described.

Fungal infections –

Gydell et al (1965) reported that disseminated histoplasmosis was seen in a 66-year-old woman on 15 mg prednisolone daily for reticulosarcoma. Non cardiosis has been observed in one patient treated for half a year with an average dose of 20 mg of prednisone for acquired haemolytic anaemia

Virus infections : An epidemic of generalized herpes zoster was observed in steroid-treated patients. Corticosteroids enhanced the susceptibility to the disease and played a part in its generalization. Severe recurrence of the herpetic eruption was observed in the course of treatment of a patient with a meningococcal meningitis with cortisone.

12) Myopathy :

Muscle weakness and atrophy can occur during treatment with steroids. There is a suggestion that the incidence of myopathy is greatest in patients being treated with a compound containing a fluorine atom in the 9a position such as triamcinolone. Myopathy may be localized especially in the muscles of the pelvic girdle. There is a lesser predilection for the shoulder girdle. Unilateral or bilateral rupture of the Achilles tendon during steroid therapy has been reported. The pain in these cases may be chronic and not very acute.

13) Withdrawal phenomena :

Long-term treatment with steroids in suppressive doses causes inhibition of corticotropin production and adrenal atrophy. Understandably acute withdrawal of the steroid dose leads to symptoms of adrenal insufficiency. The clinician should be on the alert for incipient adrenal insufficiency when symptoms of nausea, vague abdominal distress, muscle pain, diarrhoea or fever are observed. It is not always easy to decide whether such symptoms are caused by adrenal insufficiency or by recurrence of the underlying disease, that may be reactivated as the steroid dosage is tapered off.

Siegel (1965) reported a case of sudden death due to adrenal insufficiency within 2 weeks, after withdrawal of prednisone (2.5 – 5 mg daily for 1 year for asthma) .

In patients with ulcerative colitis, fever and abdominal pain developed after steroid withdrawal following colectomy that was apparently caused not by infection but by adrenal insufficiency. Sudden death following operation for ulcerative colitis has been observed in 2 cases treated with steroids preoperatively but not during and immediately after operation. Exacerbation of rheumatoid arthritis occurs when corticosteroids are withdrawn.

Several articles discuss the functional capacity of the pituitary-adrenal system after long-term treatment with corticosteroids alone or combined with ACTH. Usually the diminished adrenal reserve is reversible, often even without ACTH stimulation. However the adrenal cortex may not be able to react normally to stress for as long as 2 ½ years

15) Teeth and dentition :

Nasstrom K, Frosberg B, Petersson A et al (1985) reported a systematic study on the association between narrowing of the dental pulp chamber and the method of treatment in patients with renal diseases. The study consisted of sixty patients treated at the Department of Nephrology, University of Lund, Sweden. Twenty patients were randomly selected from each of three groups, comprising of patients who had functioning renal transplants for more than 2 years, nonuremic patients on immunosuppressive treatment, and patients on hemodialysis treatment.

As the patients had received various steroid drugs with different glucocorticoid potentials, the effects were related to that of prednisolone. Transplant patients received an average dose of 7,500 mg of prednisolone during the first year after transplantation, of which 6,200 mg was received during the first 6 months. Twelve patients had one or more episodes with transplant rejection during the first year. These rejections were treated with 1,250 to 4,000 mg of prednisolone, resulting in a total dose of prednisolone during the first year of 7,500 to 19,500 mg. During the second year, the average dose was 3,500 mg of prednisolone, and during the third year, it was 2,500 mg. the patients continuously received about 2,000 mg of prednisolone per year there-after.

The nonuremic patients on immunosuppressive treatment received an average dose of 5,000 mg of prednisolone during the first year, 4,500 mg of which was received during the first 6 months. Most of the patients continuously received about 2,000 mg of prednisolone per year thereafter. Six patients on hemodialysis treatment received prednisolone during periods of from 2 months up to 3 years before starting hemodialysis. The average dose of prednisolone in these six patients was 4,100 mg per year. The remaining nine patients on hemodialysis had not received any immunosuppressive treatment. Transplant patients and nonuremic patients under immunosuppressive treatment received about 36,500 mg of azathioprine (Immurel) yearly. Four patients (one with a transplant and three nonuremic patients) received about 21,000 mg of cyclophosphamide (Sendoxan) each during the first year after starting treatment. One of the patients continued to receive 1,800 mg of cyclophosphamide yearly. Intraoral radiographs were obtained from the patient's general dentists. Narrowing of the dental pulp chamber was studied, without the knowledge of the patient's diagnosis or treatment. Results showed that there was a strong association between narrowing of the dental pulp chamber and the method of treatment. Narrowing of the dental pulp chamber was seen in fourteen of nineteen transplant patients, in five of seventeen nonuremic patients on immunosuppressive treatment, and in two of fifteen patients on hemodialysis. There were significantly more patients with narrowing of the dental pulp chamber among the transplant patients than among nonuremic patients on immunosuppressive treatment. Patients with narrowing of the dental pulp chamber had received significantly higher doses of prednisolone than the patients without narrowing. Authors concluded that high doses of corticosteroids seem to play an important role in the initiation of this phenomenon.

Acton CHC (1986) reported a case of steroid-induced anterior open bite. Where in a young man presented with increasing anterior open bite due to severe erosion and eventual collapse of the mandibular condyles. He had been undergoing immunosuppressive treatment, including high dose prednisolone to treat the rejection of his renal transplant originally and subsequently in connection with his mitral valve replacement following infective endocarditis. He also suffered severe secondary hyperparathyroid bone disease.

Gold SI (1989) reported details of 8 year follow-up study of a patient with systemic lupus erythematosus (SLE) who was treated with up to 60 mg of prednisone per day for more than 8 years. Radiographic documentation demonstrated complete calcification of all pulp chambers and root canals during that period.

DRUG INTERACTIONS OF GLUCOCORTICOIDS

Glucocorticoid dosage is decreased :

Antibiotics (erythromycin, trioleandomycin), cyclosporine, isoniazid and ketoconazole reduce the metabolic clearance of glucocorticoids, estrogens increase the levels of corticosteroid binding protein and thus reduce the free fraction and reduce the metabolic clearance of glucocorticoids. Estrogens increase the levels of corticosteroid binding protein and thus reduce the free fraction and reduce the clearance.

Glucocorticoid dosage is increased :

Cholestyramine decreases the intestinal absorption. Antiepileptic drugs (barbiturates, phenytoin, carbamazemine), rifampicin, aminoglutothemide increase the metabolism by inducing hepatic microsomal enzymes.

Glucocorticoid dosage needs adjustment :

Antianxiety and antipsychotic drugs : Recurrent or poor control of CNS symptoms due to inherent glucocorticoid effects.

- Anticholinesterases : May precipitate myasthenic crisis.
- Anticoagulants : Effectiveness of anticoagulants decreases.
- Antihypertensives : Their effectiveness decreases.
- Hypoglycemics : Their effectiveness decreases.
- Sympathomimetics : Their effectiveness increases.
- Salicylates : Their clearance is increased.

PRECAUTIONS DURING GLUCOCORTICOID THERAPY:

These apply especially to the prolonged, high dose, suppressive therapy with glucocorticoids.

Before starting therapy :

- Enquire about and check for : peptic ulcer, diabetes mellitus, tuberculosis, any other infection (especially one not amenable to chemotherapy).

During therapy :

- Prescribe the drug with food.
- Check periodically for : weight gain, edema, hyperglycemia, hypertension, infection, GI bleeding, hypokalemia, ocular changes.
- Monitor growth in children.
- Instruct the patient not to stop the drug abruptly.
- Increase the dose in case of any stress (severe infection, major surgery).
- Prescribe oral calcium and vitamin D supplements.

While stopping therapy :

- Taper therapy

Contraindications :

There are no absolute contraindications to glucocorticoid therapy other than Cushing's syndrome and ocular herpes zoster. Proper precautions have to be taken in using them in diabetes mellitus, peptic ulcer, hypertension, CCF, osteoporosis, in debilitated or old patients and in the presence of infection.

PREPARATIONS AND DOSAGE OF GLUCO CORTICOIDS :

For systemic use :

i) Cortisone acetate (Corlin) tablets, containing 25 mg. dose : 25-37.5 mg (replacement therapy).

ii) Cortisone injection is a suspension of cortisone acetate (25 mg. per ml) in sodium chloride injection. Dose : 50 to 200 mg. daily intramuscularly in single or divided doses.

iii) Hydrocortisone tablet contains 10 mg of the drug.

iv) Hydrocortisone hemisuccinate (Efcorlin) being readily water soluble is administered intramuscularly, by intravenous infusion or as a retention enema. Approximately 133 mg of the salt contains 100 mg. of hydrocortisone. For retention enema, a dose equivalent in 120 ml of normal saline is given each night.

v) Prednisone tablet contains 5 mg of the drug, either in the pure form or as an equivalent amount of prednisone acetate. Dose : 10 to 100 mg daily in divided doses.

vi) Prednisolone tablet contains 5 mg, 10mg, 20mg & 40mg of the drug or an equivalent amount of prednisolone acetate. Dose : 10 to 100 mg daily in divided doses.

vii) Prednisolone acetate suspension contains 25 mg per ml. It is administered by intramuscular, intra-articular or peri-articular injection.

viii) Prednisolone or prednisone pediatric drops contain 5 mg of prednisolone or prednisone per ml. Dose : new-born, 0.3 to 0.4 mg per kgper dose; infants, 0.2 to 0.3 mg per kg per dose; older children, 0.15 to 0.2 mg per kg per dose.

ix) Prednisolone sodium phosphate., in contrast to prednisolone or its acetate, is soluble in water. Approximately 27 mg of the salt are equivalent to 20 mg of prednisolone. Dose : equivalent to 20-100 mg of prednisolone intravenously and 20 mg by retention enema.

x) Methylprednisolone 4 mg tablets. Dose : 2-40 mg daily individed doses.

xi) Methylprednisolone sodium succinate (Inj. Medrol). Dose : equivalent to 40-120 mg of methyl-prednisolone base by intramuscular or intravenous injection; 40 to 120 mg as a retention enema. Bolus dose 500-1000 mg of medrol.

xii) Methylprednisolone acetate injection (Depot Medrol) for I.M. use.

xiii) Triamcinolone tablet (Ledercort, Kenacort) contains 4 mg of triamcinolone. Dose : 2-24 mg daily in divided doses.

xiv) Triamcinolone diacetate injection for intramuscular or intra-articular use. Dose : 5 to 40 mg. It must not be given intravenously.

xv) Betamethasone tablet (Betnelan) contains 0.5 mg of the drug. Dose : 0.5 to 5 mg daily. For ulcerative colitis, 4 mg. twice daily in retention enema.

xvi) Betamethasone sodium phosphate, a water soluble salt is available as tablets and for injection (Betnesol); nearly 1.3 mg of the salt is equivalent to 1 mg of betamethasone. Dose : equivalent to 0.5 to 5 mg of betamethasone by mouth; for acute adrenal insufficiency, 10 to 20 mg by intravenous or intramuscular injection daily in divided doses.

xvii) Dexamethasone tablet (Decadron) contains 0.5 mg of the drug. Doses similar to betamethasone tablets.

xviii) Dexamethasone phosphate injection (Decadron injection) contains 4 mg of the salt per ml roughly 1.3 mg of the salt is equivalent to 1 mg of the base. Dose : 4 to 20 mg of the base by intramuscular or intravenous injection.

Comparison of various glucocorticoids :

Comparison of various glucocorticoids :

Drug	Biological half-life (hours)	Glucocorti - coid activity	Mineralo -corticoid activity	Suppres sion of pituitary	Compara tive doses (mg)	Affinity
Short acting						
Cortisone	8-12	0.8	1	1	25	1
Hydrocortisone	8-12	1	1.25	2.5	20	100
Intermediate acting						
Prednisolone	18-36	4	0.5	5	5	220
Methylprednisolone	18-36	5	0	8	4	1350
Triamcinolone	18-36	5	0	-	4	-
Long acting						
Dexamethasone	36-54	25	0	100-200	0.75	540
Betamethasone	36-54	25	0	100-200	0.75	400

Therapeutic uses of glucocorticoids : These can be divided into :

I. **Substitution therapy :** Addison's disease and hypopituitarism are indications for substituion therapy with glucocorticoids. They are discussed under mineralocorticoids.

II. **Pharmacological therapy :**

- **Pulse therapy :** Methylprednisolone, in i.v. bolus doses of 500-1000 mg injected slowly, once daily, for three consecutive days, is useful in threatened acute rejection of a renal graft, eye threatening Graves exophthalmos and similar dire emergencies.
- **Intensive short term therapy :** Can save life and reduce morbidity in certain potentially lethal conditions in which the inflammatory or the metabolic response of the body itself threatens life. These conditions include : allergic emergencies such as anaphylactic shock; status asthmaticus, circulatory collapse unresponsive to pressor amines, acute necrotizing vasculitis, water intoxication, central hyperthermia, and acute hypercalcemia accompanying vitamin D intoxication or hormone therapy of metastatic breast cancer. In status asthmaticus, the glucocorticoids take several hours to act and their use supplements that of the bronchodilators. In circulatory failure a single massive dose (preferably of a long acting compound) sometimes restores the blood pressure to normal.

In hypercalcemic crisis, glucocorticoids take several days to reduce the plasma calcium and must be used along with other quicker acting measures. Glucocorticoids have been shown to be effective in preventing or minimizing the long term sequelae (such as deafness) of acute bacterial meningitis, when used as adjuncts to antibiotic therapy.

In all thcsc conditions, large doses such as 100-200 mg (1-2 mg/kg/day) of prednisolone per day may have to be used but therapy with such doses seldom lasts longer than 48-72 hours. In such cases, the adverse effects of glucocorticoids mainly consists of burning and itching at the mucocutaneous junctions, and rarely of multifocal ventricular premature beats, precipitation of ketoacidotic coma in a diabetic, and acute erosive gastritis with hemorrhage.

- **Prolonged, high-dose, suppressive therapy :** is indicated in acute rheumatic fever, ulcerative colitis, celiac disease not responding to gluten-free diet, subacute hepatic necrosis, chronic active hepatitis (but not in patients positive for hepatitis B surface antigen) alcoholic hepatitis, autoimmune hemolytic anemia, idiopathic thrombocytopenic purpura, acute lymphatic leukemia, disseminated Hodgkin's disease, nephrotic syndrome, acute homograft rejection, pemphigus and collagen diseases. In these diseases, the initial dose may be as high as 100-200 mg of prednisolone per day, the therapy continues longer than 7-10 days and the maintenance dose may be 15 mg of prednisolone or more per day. The fear of adverse reactions is utmost in this group and the patients need the closest supervision. A rapid reduction in the dose can cause an acute exacerbation of the disease being treated. On the other hand, abrupt cessation is dangerous and can precipitate acute adrenocortical insufficiency. The patients must be warned about this possibility. In order to minimize the suppression of the hypothalamo-pituitary-adrenal axis during such prolonged, high-dose therapy, the alternate day regime should be tried once the clinical improvement has stabilized. If it is unable to maintain the clinical remission, the entire daily dose may be given in the morning with the same objective in mind.

- **Low-dose, chronic, palliative therapy :** Consists of the use of small doses of a glucocorticoid (2-10 mg of prednisolone per day) as an adjunct to some other drug e.g. salicylates in rheumatoid arthritis. Here, total relief of symptoms is not aimed at, in order to avoid the adverse effects of the glucocorticoid. Such low-dose therapy should not be tried on alternate days as it is ineffective in controlling the disease adequately. As the therapy is generally very prolonged, sometimes lifelong, the patients need close supervision. The dose of the glucocorticoid should be abruptly raised 2-4 times during such stress as surgery or a severe infection in such patients.

- **Chronic, suppression of pituitary ACTH secretion :** is indicated in congenital, virilizing, adrenocortical hyperplasia. This is best achieved with the use of a long acting compound such as dexamethasone or betamethasone in the dose of 0.5 mg at bedtime daily. Such therapy suppresses the urinary 17-ketosteroids adequately and rarely causes any adverse effects. It must be impressed upon the parents of such a child that the therapy must continue lifelong.

- **Topical application :** is found valuable in many dermatological, ocular and external ear conditions. Ocular conditions benefited by local corticosteroid therapy are interstitial keratitis, phlyctenular conjunctivitis, spring catarrh, iritis and iridocyclitis, whereas, posterior uveitis and sympathetic opthalmia need systemic medication.

Local steroid therapy is valuable in many inflammatory dermatoses and for controlling excerbations of pruritic eczema and psoriasis. It is not recommended for urticaria.

Unfortunately, steroid ointments are being misused as a dermatological panacea because they usually give dramatic relief in inflammatory and pruritic conditions of the skin.

Their indiscriminate use, however, is not only wasteful but also harmful. Application of a steroid ointment for such conditions as herpes simplex, herpes zoster, ringworm and impetigo may lead to marked exacerbation of the disease.

Corticosteroids accelerate the fungal growth and spread, and cause local skin atrophy with resultant telangiectasia, purpura and striae.

Further, systemic toxicity including adrenal suppression can occur following local corticosteroid therapy, more so in infants; and hence, potent preparations like betamethasone valerate, triamcinolone acetonide, fluocinolone acetonide and clobetasol propionate should not be prescribed for treating infantile eczema.

Similarly such potent steroids should not be applied to facial skin as atrophy and telangiectasia occur more quickly on the face.

The current practice of adding a glucocorticoid to antibiotics and antifungal agents is difficult to justify. The same is true of use of glucocorticoids in ointments for hemorrhoids.

TOPICAL STEROIDS :

Topical corticosteroids possess antiinflammatory and antimitotic activity and are the cornerstone of treatment for many inflammatory skin and mucosal conditions.

They are classified according to vasoconstrictor assay (classes 1 through 7) or clinical efficacy (five groupings) in alleviating signs and symptoms of inflammatory dermatoses. Topical steroids are absorbed at different rates from different parts of the body.

For example, the rate of absorption from the eyelids and genitals is 30%, 7% from the face, 1% from the forearm, and 0.1% from the palm. The lowest, potency steroid should be selected and used for the shortest possible time.

Lower potency steroids should be used on more sensitive areas such as the face, eyelids, and groin, whereas more potent agents are used on thicker skinned areas such as the palms and soles.

Topical steroids are available in cream, ointment, gel and liquid vehicles. When comparing different forms of the same steroid preparation, ointments are generally stronger than creams because they penetrate better and are absorbed best.

Steroids that are used on the oral mucosa are prepared in orabase dental paste.

Common skin and mucosal lesions that may be treated with topical steroids :

Skin lesions	**Lesions of oral mucosa**
Atopic dermatitis (eczema)	Oral Crohn's disease, Lichen planus
Psoriasis	Desquamative gingivitis
Seborrheic dermatitis	Recurrent aphthous stomatitis, oral presentation of lupus erythematosus, Small traumatic oral ulcers chapped or cracked lips

Topical steroid preparations : potency and available forms :

Potency	Drug	Forms
Low	Fluocinolone acetonide (Synlar) 0.01% Hydrocortisone 0.25%, 0.5%, 1%, 2.5%	C, S C, O
Medium	Betamethasone benzoate (Uticort) 0.025% Desonide (desOwen) 0.05% Dexamethasone (Decadron) 0.1% Fluocinolone (Synlar) 0.025% Triamcinolone (Kenalog) 0.025%	C, G C C C, O C, O
Medium high	Betamethasone valerate (Valisone) 0.1% Dexamethasone elixir (Decadron) 0.5% Triamcinolone (Kenalog) 0.1%	C S C,O
High	Halcinonide (Halog) 0.1% Fluocinonide (Lidex) 0.05% Flucinolone acetonide (Synlar) 0.2% Triamcinolone (Kenalog) 0.5%	C, O C, O, G, S C C, O
Super high	Betamethasone diproprionate augmented (Diprolene) 0.05% Clobetasol (Temovate) 0.05% Halobetasol proprionate (Ultravate) 0.05%	O C, O, G C, O

C = cream, O = ointment, G = Gel, S = solution

Adverse effects of topical cortiocosteroids may be local or systemic. Common local effects are skin atrophy (thinning), striae, telangiectasia, hypopigmentation, perioral dermatitis, acneform eruption and hypersensitivity reactions. Care should be taken when prescribing topical steroids for use on the facial skin of young children because it may cause problems. Their skin may become permanently reddened (or bleached in the case of black children) or it may atrophy. Systemic side effects also may occur more readily in young children. High potency steroids are not recommended for routine topical use in children.

Systemic effects of topical steroids depend on several factors such as the amount of steroid applied, the surface area covered, the site treated, the nature of the skin or mucosal problem (inflammation or other disease processes in the skin or mucosa increase percutaneous absorption), application frequency, the length of time of application, potency of the steroid, and vehicle formation.

When large amounts of steroids are absorbed through the skin, fluid retention, raised blood pressure, and secondary diabetes may develop or it may aggravate these conditions in patients already under therapy. Suppression of the hypothalamic-pituitary-adrenal axis with the use of topical steroids is uncommon in adults, however, can occur when more potent agents are used excessively.

Adrenal suppression caused by topical steroid use is seen more frequently in small children because their body surface area is large relative to their total body weight.

Once absorbed through the skin, topical corticosteroids are handled through pharmocokinetc pathways similar to systemically administered corticosteroids. They are metabolized primarily in the liver and are excreted by the kidneys.

For dermatologic use the least potent steroid should be used for the shortest period of time. These steroid preparations are all similar in function and differ primarily by the strength of each compound. They decrease local inflammation, swelling, burning and itching. Ointment forms help to maintain skin moisture, whereas creams are useful in open, moist skin lesions. The authors have found topical steroid creams to be useful after long intraoral surgery that results in excessive trauma (from retraction) to the lip commissure and its adjacent skin. The major contraindications are systemic fungal infections, other infections, and hypersensitivity to the drug.

Kenalog in orabase :

This steroid is a 0.1% triamcinolone acetonide preparation specially formulated for intraoral use. Each gram of the paste provides 1 mg of triamcinolone acetonide. It is indicated for the treatment of ulcerative diseases, as adjunctive therapy for the temporary relief of symptoms associated with oral inflammatory lesions, and for ulcerations that result from trauma.

It is used by placing a small amount (0.25 inch length dispensed from the tube) to the lesion until a thin film develops. Only enough of paste to cover the lesion with a thin film should be used and it should not be rubbed. It should be used two to three times per day, preferably after breakfast and lunch and then at bedtime, with bedtime application being the most important.

Contraindications are hypersensitivity to the drug, fungal, viral, or bacterial infections of the mouth or throat, active tuberculosis, uncontrolled diabetes, and pregnancy.

Another similar, less potent agent is orabase HCA (hydrocortisone acetate 0.5%.

Addy M, Pimlott SJ, Thaw M (1986) compared the oral retention of prednisolone sodium phosphate with prednisolone alcohol and measured the effects of time and concentration upon such retention in normal healthy volunteers.

A total of 14 subjects (8 male, 6 female) of age range 20-34 years were selected for the study.

Staff and student volunteers were selected on the basis of being dentate, without partial dentures and free from oral ulceration. The subjects had a good standard of oral hygiene and periodontal health. In view of the number of proposed rinses, volunteers were randomly allocated to two groups to which four rinsing regimens were assigned as follows:

Group A PSP – 250,500 and 1000 μg/ml solution rinsed for 5 minutes and 500 μg/ml solution rinsed for 2 minutes.

Group B PSP – 100 and 500 μg/ml solution rinsed for 5 mintues and PA 100 and 500 μg/ml solution rinsed for 5 minutes.

Volunteers in each group repeated each of their four regimens three times.

Four of the volunteers in the study were randomly selected to provide samples of unstimulated mixed whole saliva. The difference between the optical density of PSP containing saliva and distilled water containing saliva was compared with the optical density of the diluted drug solution which contained no saliva.

Results showed that for groups A and B, the percentage of the dose retained after rinsing was essentially similar for all, but the 100μg/ml rinse, where the percentage retention was significantly increased to 30% of the dose delivered.

The results demonstrated that if PSP were to be used as a mouthrinse in the oral cavity, doses will be retained from higher concentration solutions. Unfortunately, 85% - 90% of the total dose would still be expectorated. A relatively longer rinsing time of 5 minutes appears to offer no advantage over a more acceptable time of 2 minutes.

Brook IM, Van Noort R, Pandurangi AV et al (1991) reported the development and initial in vivo testing of a device suitable for controlled intraoral delivery of hydrocortisone sodium succinate (HSS).

Disks of polymethyl methacrylate (PMMA) loaded with HSS, 32% wt/wt, were produced by mixing HSS (molecular weight 484 daltons; Glaxo Laboratories, Middlesex, U.K), supplied as an off-white powder, with PMMA beads before being added to methyl methacrylate (MMA) monomer (Simplex Rapid Clear, Howmedica International, London, U.K.). The mix was vigorously spatulated and poured into flexible molds. Curing was undertaken in a palamat hydroflask (Kulzer and Co. gmbH, Friedrichsdorf, Germany) at 55^0C and at 3.5 atm pressure for 20 minutes. These disks, which formed the core of the device, were modified to control the release of drug by partial coating with drug-free PMMA and the addition of a semipermeable membrane (SPM) to the remaining surface.

Release of drug from devices with and without SPM was undertaken into a glass of distilled water at 37^0C for 7 days by a method reported previously. Before in vitro testing, six disks were selected at random from the same batch as used in the volunteers, and the in vitro release rate for the batch was determined. Immediately after sampling, analysis of the amount of drug released was undertaken with a Cecil CE 595 double-beam digital UV / visible light spectrophotometer (Cecil Instrumetns Ltd., Cambridge, U.K.) set at the maximum absorbance for HSS of 248 nm.

Five male volunteers, certified as fit to participate in the trial by their own general medical practitioner and who were taking no concommitant medication, were entered into the study. For each a holding plate was constructed to hold the device, which was nominally 9 mm in diameter and 3 mm thick and contained 65 mg of HSS.

Saliva was sampled twice a day, at 8 AM before breakfast and at 6 PM before dinner, from Sunday to Sunday. Holding plates containing the drug-releasing device were placed in the mouth after the 8 AM Monday Sampling. They were maintained in the mouth until after the 6 PM sample on Saturday and were removed only while eating or when cleaning the teeth.

For comparison with an intermittent dosing regimen, 1 week after the study of the intraoral devices, the same volunteers took a single dose (2.5 mg) of HSS (Corlan lozenge). Saliva samples were then obtained at 10-, 20-, 40-, 60-, 80- and 100- minute intervals.

Except for subject / other subjects were able to wear the holders without complications and reported a mild bitter taste, which was more noticeable in the mornings, correlating with the higher salivary levels of HSS at this time. While the devices were being worn, morning HSS saliva levels were maintained at a mean (±SD) of approximately 49 (± 13 mg/L); the evening levels were significantly lower (Student's t test; $t = 4.48$, $df = 6$, $p < 0.005$) but were maintained at a mean (±SD) of approximately 19 (± 6 mg/L), which did not decay toward the end of the test period.

The devices, were able to maintain consistent morning and evening levels during the 6-day period, and release did not decay with time. Further work into the time it takes for a therapeutic level to be established and indeed the therapeutic level actually required is needed.

- **Intra-articular and intratendinous use :** Long acting esters of glucocorticoids have been used successfully to treat painful osteoarthritis and painful tender fascial nodules by local infiltration. Such therapy has the added advantage of minimum systemic absorption and consequent reduction in toxicity.
- **Diagnostic tests :** Dexamethasone suppression of adrenal function; cortisone test in hypercalcemia; and prednisolone test to distinguish intra and extra hepatic obstructive jaundice.
- **Miscellaneous :** Glucocorticoids have been used in a wide variety of other conditions which includes Bell's palsy, acute infective polyneuritis, encephalitis,

infective hepatitis, complete heart block, hyperarrhythmia and so on. Their usefulness in the therapy of these conditions is doubtful.

They can be life saving in cerebral edema due to neoplasms, particularly metastases. Usually, dexamethasone is injected in the dose of 8 mg., 6-8 hourly. Their value in cerebral edema due to head injury and stroke is unproven. Other measures used to reduce cerebral edema are intravenous furosemide (40-60 mg) mannitol (1 g per kg) or urea (1 g per kg., 30% sol); oral administration of pure glycerine (15-30 ml thrice daily) and rectal administration of saturated magnesium sulfate solution (50-200 ml).

MANAGEMENT OF DENTAL PATIENTS TAKING CORTICOSTEROIDS :

Patients receiving glucocorticoids in doses greater than the equivalent of 30 mg. of cortisone daily for a continuous period of one week or longer have a possibility of developing adrenal crisis. Persons who have discontinued this type of therapy within the past year are also at risk. The higher the daily dosage, longer the period of administration, or shorter the period since discontinuation, greater is the potential risk of adrenal crisis.

Since adrenal crisis is due to the patient's inability to produce sufficient amounts of endogenous cortisol in response to stress, all efforts should be made to minimize the degree of anxiety experienced. In addition to anxiety control, blood glucocorticoid levels must be increased prior to a stressful situation. This can be accomplished through administration of a “steroid prep”. A steroid prep is a controlled increase of glucocorticoids given prior to the patient’s dental appointment which is slowly reduced to a normal dosage level over a 2 to 3 day period following therapy. Failure to use a schedule of gradual reduction can result in iatrogenic adrenal insufficiency, which can cause collapse and death.

Several regimens of management for the risk patient during dental therapy have been suggested. Most are nonspecific or tend to underestimate the degree of stress associated with dental treatment.

Dentists must carefully evaluate the extent of dental procedures and estimate the apprehension of patients prior to discussing their recommendations with physicians. The following guidelines may be used to categorize management :

I. A) Routine noninvasive dental therapy (examination, impressions, etc.)

B) A nonapprehensive patient

C) Slight risk of pituitary-adrenal suppression.

- No steroid prep is required.
- Light sedation is optional.

II. A) Routine invasive dental therapy (restorations, routine endodontics, scaling and root planning, biopsy)

B) A moderately apprehensive patient

C) Relatively greater risk of pituitary-adrenal suppression.

- A steroid prep consisting of doubling the daily dosage of glucocorticoid prior to the procedure followed by gradually reducing the dose each day for 3 days back to the normal dosage.

- Light to moderate sedation.

III. A) Combination of two or three factors from Category II

B) Extensive invasive dental therapy (long restorative or endodontic procedures, multiple extractions, periodontal or endodontic surgery)

C) An extremely apprehensive patient

D) Severe risk of pituitary-adrenal suppression.

- A steroid preparation consisting of quadrupling the daily dosage of glucocorticoid prior to the procedure followed by gradual reduction over a 2- or 3- day period to the normal dosage.

- Moderate to heavy sedation.

IV. Combination of two or more of the situations in category III or a long surgical procedure.

- Hospitalization of the patient where administration of extensive doses of glucocorticoids, heavy sedation, and appropriate monitoring can be provided.

All administration of steroid preps should be by mutual agreement with the physician in charge of glucocorticoid therapy. If there is doubt about how to manage the patient, one should choose the most rigorous protocol. It is safer to overadminister prophylactic steroid preps than to underadminister the same.

Ronald LTC, Butter CD, Vorono AA et al (1993) conducted a study to determine the effects of two dosage regimen of dexamethasone on the serum cortisol levels of a group of patients undergoing major maxillofacial surgical procedures. They concluded that the use of dexamethasone, 10 to 20 mg intravenously given every 3 hours intraoperatively and every 4 hours postoperatively over 24 hours, followed by a repository dose of 80 mg of intramuscular methylprednisolone, causes short term serum cortisol suppression. The maximum depression occurred on postoperatively day 3, normal levels were restored by postoperative day 7. Therefore, pulsed therapy can be considered relatively safe when known contraindications have been considered.

Miller CS, Dembo JB, Falace DA (1995) conducted a study with the intent of determining the level of stress displayed by healthy patients who underwent five types of routine dental treatment (examination, prophylaxis, restoration, root canal therapy, extraction) by analyzing salivary levels of cortisol before, during, and after the operation. It was anticipated that these data would help in the formulation of guidelines for the dental treatment of patients with secondary adrenal insufficiency. The physiologic stress of various dental procedures was measured in 50 nonsmoking healthy men between the ages of 18 and 55 years with a salivary cortisol assay.

The physiologic stress of various dental procedures (dental examination, dental prophylaxis, restoration, root canal therapy, and tooth extraction) was measured in 50 nonsmoking healthy men between the ages of 18 and 55 years (mean 34.6 years, range 21 to 53 years) with a salivary cortisol assay. Expectorated saliva was collected at four time points: 10 minutes before the start of the procedure, 15 minutes after the patient was seated, at the end of the procedure, and 1 hour after the completion of the procedure. Of the 196 samples included for analysis, mean cortisol values ranged from 0.1 to 3.8μg/dl with a recovery of 100%±8.4%. The mean cortisol value for the extraction group (1.09±0.42μg/dl) was significantly different ($p<0.05$) from the mean values of the examination (0.46 ±0.10 μg/dl), prophylaxis (0.64±0.64μg/dl), root canal (0.49±0.07 μg/dl), and restorative (0.60±0.04μg/dl) groups as determined by the Duncan's multiple range test. Cortisol levels decreased from the initial reading to the end of the procedure by about 15% for patients undergoing an examination, root canal, and restorative procedure. Cortisol levels at the end of the procedure were elevated in the prophylaxis (55%) and extraction (148%) groups compared with the baseline cortisol recording. A minority of patients in the prophylaxis group had elevated cortisol levels throughout dental treatment, whereas cortisol levels were elevated during treatment in 80% of patients undergoing extraction. These data suggest that the adrenal stress response associated with tooth extraction(s) is greater than that associated with other routine dental procedure.

Thomason JM et al (1999) conducted a randomized, crossover, double-blind trial to determine whether organ transplant patients requiring gingival surgery need supplementary corticosteroid cover. 20 organ transplant patients (18 male and 2 female) with clinically significant drug-induced gingival overgrowth in at least 2 quadrants of their mouth agreed to participate in the study. All patients were medicated with cyclosporin and prednisolone for at least months prior to the gingival surgery. All gingivectomies were scheduled for the first half of the morning. All patients were operated upon in the first half of the morning. Prior to gingival surgery, resting blood pressure (BP) and serum ACTH concentrations were determined. Immediately before surgery patients received either intravenous hydrocortisone 100 mg or placebo in random, double-blind order. Each patient required 2 gingivectomies and thus acted as their own control. BP was measured at various time points throughout the surgery and upto 2 hrs postoperatively. On completion of surgery, a further blood sample was taken to determine ACTH concentration. There was no significant difference between effects of placebo and hydrocortisone administration on BP and ACTH measurements. No patient experienced any symptoms that were suggestive of adrenocortical suppression. One patient did experience postural hypotension prior to gingival surgery, but this was attributed to his antidepressant medication. They conclude from this study that immunosuppressed organ transplant patients taking the maintenance dose of prednisolone (5-10 mg/day) do not require supplemental corticosteroid cover prior to gingival surgery under local anaesthesia. However, advocate monitoring of their blood pressure throughout the procedure was advocated.

USES IN DENTISTRY :

USES IN ORAL MEDICINE

- Lichen planus
- Oral submucous fibrosis
- Aphthous stomatitis
- Pemphigus
- Bell's palsy
- Mucocele
- Psoriasis
- Erythema multiforme
- Herpes virus infection
- Central giant cell granuloma
- Temporomandibular joint pain and dysfunction
- Chronic ulcerative stomatitis
- Pystomatitis vegetans
- Giant haemangioma
- Meischer's granulomatous cheilitis

USES IN ORAL SURGERY :

- Third molar surgery
- Reconstructive oral surgery
- Preprosthetic surgery
- Adjunctive use

USE IN ENDODONTICS

ORAL MEDICINE :

Introduction :

Glucocorticosteroids are used in oral medicine because of their anti-inflammatory and immunosuppressive effects. As immunity and inflammation work together in body defense, the anti-inflammatory and immuno-suppressive effects of steroids together regulate these defense reactions.

LICHEN PLANUS

Lichen planus is a common chronic inflammatory disease of the skin and oral mucosa. The erosive type of oral lichen planus can be particularly painful and may interfere with eating, speaking and swallowing. Long-standing erosive and atrophic oral lichen planus can in a few instance be transformed into squamous cell carcinoma. Although the etiology of lichen planus is still unknown, there are indications that it may be associated with stress, some systemic diseases, drugs and immunologic disorders. Various new treatments have recently been tried but complete cure is difficult. Corticosteroids have been widely used for reducing inflammation and pain and remain the management of choice.

Zegarelli DJ (1983) conducted a study to describe three therapeutic modalities of delivering steroid medication to the lesions of twenty patients and utilizing these different modalities in multiple form in order to obtain maximum benefit.

Twenty patients with one or more intraoral erosive / ulcerative LP lesions were selected in sequence and serve as the subjects of this report. In addition to clinical evidence of erosive / ulcerative LP lesions each case was documented microscopically according to Shklar's histologic criteria.

Fifteen patients were female and five were male. Each patient was given steroids in a multiple administrative manner, namely : 1) topical and injectable ; or 2) topical and systemic ; or 3) topical, injectable and systemic. The methodology of each regimen was as follows.

1) Topical and injectable: The topical steroid Kenalog in Orabase (triamcinolone acetonide in orabase) was applied to the affected sites as a thin film, Q.I.D. after meals and before sleep for at least three weeks. During this same period one or more erosive / ulcerative lesions were injected with methyl prednisolone once a week for 1 or 2 or 3 weeks depending upon the size of the lesion, its severity and the tissue response. A 27 gauge, 2 ml disposable tuberculin syringe was used to inject the steroid submucosally, parallel to and just beneath the lesion's surface. Methylprednisolone 40mg/ml (Depo-Medrol 40) was used injecting from 0.3 to 1.0 ml per lesion. In some cases a local anesthetic was administered prior to steroid injection in order to avoid undue discomfort.

1) Topical and systemic : The topical steroid was administered as describe above. The systemic steroid prednisone, was administered in the following manner : 30

mg per day for the first week, 15 mg per day for the second, and 5 mg per day for the third and final week of treatment.

2) Topical, injectable and systemic: All three modalities as described above were utilized in treating this group of patients.

All patients were required to return for follow-up observation, injection of steroid, and adjustment of medication where necessary, at least one a week. A zero response indicated no improvement ; a 25% improvement was used to denote minimal improvement, consisting of mild subjective relief and a small reduction in lesion size. A 50% improvement consisted of a moderate resolution of the lesion and obvious subjective improvement ; A 75% improvement was used when most of the lesion had disappeared and where dramatic subjective improvement was noted. A 100% response meant that there was complete or almost complete disappearance of the lesions and subjectively the patient was pain-free.

Seven patients received the topical and injectable regimen, five followed the topical and systemic regimen, and eight received the topical, injectable and systemic regimen.

1) Topical and injectable : Five of these seven were graded as having a 100% clinical improvement ; one patient had a 75% improvement and one was considered 25% or merely mild improvement. One patient after treatment developed increased lesional keratinization which is typical of reticular LP.

In most cases, where recurrence did appear, they did so only after many months of comfort and furthermore, topical therapy alone was successful in adequately controlling the lesions.

Vincent SD et al (1990) reviewed the clinical and historic features of 100 patients referred to their clinic for diagnosis and management of lichen planus. The age, gender, chief complaint, duration of the chief complaint, medical history, medications and clinical findings were recorded. Past therapeutic modalities were reviewed.

Oral lichen planus responded most favourably to treatment with topical or systemic steroids. The decision to use topical steroid, systemic steroid, or a combination of both is based on professional judgement. In this study topical regimen for diffuse oral lesions consisted of a 0.1% or 0.2% triamcinolone acetonide aqueous suspension.

Patients were advised to rinse with 5ml four times per day, after meals and at bedtime, and to take nothing by mouth for at least 1 hour after rinsing.

In cases showing significant clinical ulceration, authors often supplement the topical triamcinolone with a short therapeutic burst regimen of systemic steroids. The usual regimen consists of 40mg of prednisone 1.5 hours after arising for 5 consecutive days, followed by a 10 to 20mg dose 1.5 hours after arising every other morning for an additional 2 weeks.

Seventeen patients in the study were treated with an initial combination of burst systemic prednisone and topical 0.1% or 0.2% topical triamcinolone acetonide.

One patient required an intralesional steroid injection to promote healing of a localized ulcer resistant to healing after topical and systemic steroid usage. 10 to 20mg of injectable triamcinolone acetonide diluted with 0.5ml with sterile water for injection & lidocaine 2% to treat chronic ulcers that show little or no evidence of healing over 2 to 6 weeks was used.

They concluded that for patients with symptoms, the use of topical aqueous triamcinolone acetonide suspension was effective in reducing mucosal erythema and ulceration. In some cases, an initial burst of systemic steroid therapy was necessary to control the ulcers and erythema, but continued remission of the oral symptoms was usually maintained adequately with use of the topical regimen alone.

Plemons JM, Zachariah NY (1990) : The objective of this study was to attempt to quantitate the amount of steroid absorbed systemically through the oral mucosa in patients who use these drugs in the management of their oral desquamative diseases. In addition, serum and urine cortisol levels were measured to evaluate potential adrenal suppression as is often encountered during steroid therapy. Systemic absorption and adrenal suppression were also evaluated in normal patients who applied the same topical steroid so that comparisons with the diseased patients could be made.

Ten patients with biopsy confirmation of erosive lichen planus volunteered for participation in the study. In addition, eight patients without oral lesions were selected to serve as controls. Each patient denied the use of topical or systemic steroids over the previous 6 months.

The detection of fluocinonide absorption and excretion was attempted by high-pressure liquid chromatography (HPLC). Serum and urine cortisol levels were measured by means of radioimmunoassay (RIA).

Ten patients with erosive lichen planus and eight control patients provided urine and blood samples at baseline, day 3, and day 21. After establishment of baseline laboratory values, patients were instructed to apply 500mg of a 0.05% fluocinonide gel to the gingiva and buccal mucosa three times a day for 3 weeks. None of the patients showed evidence of systemic absorption of the steroid during the study.

The results showed that during the 3 weeks of topical administration fluocinonide, these patients demonstrated partial remission of their oral lesions.

Urine cortisol levels showed no evidence of change that might indicate adrenal suppression.

Although the detection of fluocinonide was possible with the use of high-pressure liquid chromatography, it was not detected in the urine of any of the patients at any of the three time periods. However, the control and spiked specimens consistently revealed fluocinonide peaks.

Study showed that adrenal suppression did not occur subsequent to the topical application of a controlled amount of fluocinonide containing gel to the gingiva and buccal mucosa of patients with erosive lichen planus or in healthy control patients over a period of 3 weeks. In addition, patients with erosive lichen planus did not appear to be more likely to have adrenal suppression under the conditions of this investigation than healthy control patients despite alterations in the continuity of their oral epithelium.

Boyd AS, Neldner KH (1991) stated that oral or systemic administration of corticosteroids is useful in relieving pruritus and in inducing a remission.

The minimal effective dose of daily prednisone used to treat patients with LP is usually 15 to 20mg. Treatment is continued for 6 weeks and then gradually tapered for another 6 weeks.

For limited involvement topical corticosteroid preparations may suffice. Occlusion overnight with polyethylene film is useful. Vulvar involvement often responds to topical applications of corticosteroids. Vaginal or rectal cortisone suppositories inserted intravaginally are helpful. One percent hydrocortisone cream as a lubricant, with regular vaginal dilator use, may prevent vaginal synechiae.

With oral lesions ointments tend to be the most helpful because gels may irritate and creams are often bitter. Steroid ointment-covered pledgets inserted intraoraly for several minutes have been recommended. Betamethasone valerate inhalers are effective in oral disease, and the lozenge form is used to treat esophageal involvement.

Intralesional triamcinolone acetonide has been injected into the affected matrices of patients with nail involvement. Both cutaneous and oral lesions respond well to intralesional steroids.

They concluded that the establishment of more rigid clinicopathologic criteria would help to clarify the cause, natural history, and treatment of the various manifestations of this common reaction pattern. Once the nosologic position of a given patient can be determined, the preferred treatment and the prognosis should be much easier and far more accurate than is now possible.

Silverman S et al (1991) conducted a study, to update and compare clinical findings in a current and previously unreported group of patients with OLP treated, and followed in oral medicine clinics during the past 5 years.

Two hundred fourteen adult patients with a clinical and biopsy-confirmed diagnosis of lichen planus were prospectively followed up.

The patients were categorized into one of three clinical forms of lichen planus : reticular, atrophic (reticular keratosis with an erythematous mucosa), and a form with reticular and atrophic features accompanied with mucosal ulceration. All patients were followed up for a minimum of 6 months to qualify for the study.

All patients were offered topical or systemic treatment, or both.

Initial treatment included either daily use of 0.05% fluocinonide (Lidex) ointment mixed with equal parts Orabase paste (applied five to ten times each day) or peroral prednisone (swallowed as 20mg tablets two to three times each day).

Results showed that the family histories of lichen planus were extremely rare. There were no evident associations with drug use, systemic diseases, tobacco use, or the presence of fungi.

Most patients had multiple sites of involvement, with the buccal mucosa being the most common site. No gender differences related to sites were evident.

Sixty-nine patients with moderate to severe pain were initially treated with either systemic or topical corticosteroids. Their pain control was gauged within 2 weeks after initiation of treatment by a visual analog scale. Almost all patients showed at least a 50% improvement. Most patients required continued intermittent corticosteroid treatment to control the discomfort of their disease.

Because OLP is not a curable condition, treatment is administered for symptoms of discomfort or pain. Treatment can involve the administration of systemic and / or topical medications. Because OLP is a T-lymphocyte mediated disease, corticosteroids are reproducibly the most effective modality of treatment. When systemic corticosteroids are used, short-term, high-dosage (prednisone 40 to 60mg/day for < 2 weeks) is the most effective form. Although topical corticosteroids also can be effective for initial treatment, they are extremely helpful in maintaining a level of control compatible with a good quality of life for many patients. In addition to the fluocinonide paste used in this study, 0.05% clobetasol (tenovate) ointment mixed with equal parts Orabase paste has also been effective.

When systemic corticosteroids are indicated and potential adverse side effects are anticipated because of preexisting medical conditions. The effective dose of corticosteroids can be reduced by combining a lower-dose form with a synergistic cytotoxic drug such as azathioprine. Topical corticosteroid mouth rinses also can be helpful in the initial treatment or in maintenance of remission of oral lichen planus.

Thongprasom K, Laungjarmekorn L, Sererat T, Taweesap W (1992) compared the topical steroid, fluocinolone acetonide in orabase (FAO) at the concentration of 0.1% for the treatment of oral lichen planus (OLP) with Triamcinolone acetonide (TAO) 0.1%. They also investigated for possible systemic and local adverse effects by smear for candida albicans, peripheral blood lymphocyte and eosinophil counts, blood pressure, and plasma cortisol assay.

Forty patients with erosive and atrophic oral lichen planus confirmed by tissue biopsy were studied.

Twenty cases were treated with 0.1% TAO in orabase and the other twenty cases with 0.1% FAO in orabase. Patients were advised to apply the FAO or TAO topically to the lesions four times a day for 1 month. The comparisons of treatment between the FAO and TAO groups were evaluated after wk 2 and wk 4.

They reported that the comparison of OLP patients treated with the TAO and the FAO after wk 2 and wk 4 indicated that there was no statistically significant clinical improvement between the two groups at 2 wk but, after 4 wk, the lesions in 13 of 19 cases in the FAO group were cured whereas the lesions in only 8 of 19 cases in the TAO were cured.

There was a statistically significant difference after 4 wk treatment in the FAO and TAO groups.

From this study it was concluded that there were no differences in blood pressure, plasma cortisol or number of circulating lymphocytes after treatment with FAO, but the number of eosinophils was reduced in every case after treatment for 6 months. There was no permanent adrenal cortical suppression after treatment for 6 months. Acute pseudomembranous candidiasis during the treatment was common but could be cured with antifungal drug in every case. This study showed that FAO in majority of cases is an effective treatment of oral lichen planus without any serious clinical side effects apart from treatable candidiasis.

Voute BEA et al (1993) conducted a randomized, double-blind, and placebo-controlled trial with the drug or placebo applied to the lesions of the oral mucosa for a period of 9 weeks. Forty consecutive patients with symptoms of oral lichen planus were seen. Twenty patients received the fluuocinonide ointment and 20 patients received the placebo.

The drug under study was fluocinonide (Topsyne fatty ointment) 1:1 homogenously incorporated in an adhesive ointment base that contained 40% hypromellose in white soft paraffin. The resulting concentration was 0.025% wt / wt of fluocinonide. The Topsyne ointment also contained wool fat derivative 5% (A merchol CAB). Propylene carbonate 3.5% propylene glycol 1.5% petrolatum ultima 36%, and white soft paraffin 54%.

At this first visit, the participants were instructed how to apply the ointment on dried lesions at least six times a day. They were instructed not to eat or drink for 30 minutes afterwards.

They reported that with respect to signs in the group of patients who received the drug, four patients (20%) showed complete response and 12 patients (60%) showed a good or partial response to the topical ointment. In the placebo group, these figures were 0 (0%) and 6 (30%), respectively. The majority of the placebo group (70%) did not respond at all. In the fluocinonide group, only four patients (20%) did not respond to therapy.

The difference in results between the fluocinonide group and placebo group was statistically significant with regard to signs (x_t^2=10.4, p=0.0013).

They concluded that topical application of fluocinonide in an adhesive base is a safe and effective therapy to reduce signs and symptoms in oral lichen planus.

Lozada-Nur F et al (1994) conducted a randomized, double-blind clinical trial to compare 0.05% clobetasol 17-propionate, a potent topical steroid, and 0.05% fluocinonide ointment, a lesspotent topical steroid, for their effectiveness in controlling oral vesiculobullous diseases (OVBD), as measured by relief of symptoms, complete disease control, longer remission time after therapy is discontinued, and minimal adverse side effects.

The drug clobetasol 17-propionate ointment contained clobetasol propionate 0.5mg/gm in a base of propylene glycol, sorbitol sesquioleate, and white petrolatum.

The ointments were mixed with orabase, equal parts by weight of the adhesive paste and 0.05% fluocinonide or 0.05% clobetasol propionate.

Sixty patients with clinical and biopsy-proven OVBD were asked to participate. There were 43 women and 17 men patients; 35 patients had lichen planus, 3 patients had benign mucous membrane pemphigoid, 3 patients had vulgaris, and 19 patients had erythema multiforme. Fifty-five patients completed the study.

Instructions called for three applications a day-after breakfast, after dinner, and before bedtime-for a total of 14 days.

The study lasted a total of 28 days, but the topical steroids were used for 14 days.

They showed that the group who used topical clobetasol propionate tended to show greater improvement beginning the first week in comparison with the group using fluocinonide ; however, the differences between the means of the two groups were not statistically significant. For erythema, atrophy, and ulcer size, 75% of the observations showed improvement in each group.Pain control was achieved by both drugs, but the group who used clobetasol showed greater improvement in the first and second weeks. Control of pain was maintained with clobetasol up to 3 weeks after therapy was discontinued.

Of the 55 lesions, 8 (14%) cleared completely after 1 week of therapy and 12 (21%) cleared completely after 2 weeks of therapy. In all, 20 (36%) of the target lesions (20% clobetasol group, 16% fluocinonide group) cleared completely during the treatment period. There was no pronounced differences between the two drugs in time or degree of clinical resolution.

Topical steroids, when used as described in this article for the treatment of OVBD, remain a safe and clinically effective treatment modality for severe chronic OVBD. The differences in response observed for pain, together with data obtained by use of the vasoconstrictor assay, clearly demonstrate the greater benefits and potency of clobetasol over fluocinonide. This finding could suggest that less severe disease will respond to the use of a topical steroid whereas severe symptomatic disease will respond sooner to a high-potency steroid at least initially. In addition, the longer remission observed in the clobetasol group – up to 3 weeks after therapy was discontinued – may indicate that better control initially can result in a longer remission.

Lu S, Chen WJ, Eng HL (1995) conducted a clinical trial to assess the benefits and clinical efficacy of the combination of prednisolone and levamisole in the treatment of OLP.

Twenty-three patients with OLP composed the study group.

Levamisole was administered 50mg three times a day and prednisolone administered 5mg three times a day for 3 consecutive days per week were used as long as evidence of relief from symptomatic OLP was seen. Patients were monitored once a week for the first 2 months and once a month thereafter for recording of clinical responses and side effects.

They revealed that 12 patients showed a dramatic response and 11 showed a partial response of signs and symptoms within 2 weeks. Almost all exhibited a dramatic response after the whole treatment course of 4 to 6 weeks was complete and remained completely free from symptoms of disease from 6 to 9 months without any additional medication.

The time of response after initiation of therapy ranged from 1 to 4 weeks before effective clinical control was achieved. All patients showed marked improvement with resolution of erosions and ulcers.

A tentative conclusion of this pilot study was that levamisole appeared to alter the course of OLP treated with systemic prednisolone. The authors found that this corticosteroid-sparing, combination drug approach for patients with OLP seems to produce clinical control with diminution of the side effects related to long term, high-dosage prednisolone.

Gorsky M et al (1996) evaluated the natural history of OLP in a group of Israeli Jews, to assess its risk of malignant transformation, and to indicate, generally, its similarity to studies conducted in other populations.

A total of 157 Jewish patients (95 women and 62 men) with histologically confirmed clinical diagnosis of OLP were studied.

The degree of symptoms at the first clinical visit was established with a linear method.

Patients with symptoms were treated with either systemic or topical corticosteroids, and all patients were monitored for a minimum of 3 months up to 15 years with a mean time of 1.5years. Forty-eight patients were monitored for approximately 6 months ; most patients were monitored for 6 months up to 3 years. Only 3% were monitored for more than 7 years.

There were more women with OLP than men. No evident association of diabetes ($p>0.50$) or cardiovascular diseases ($p=0.10$) was found (22%). All the patients had either skin lesions of lichen planus or a documented history of skin involvement.

A positive Candida culture was observed in 32% of the entire group with no specific predilection to clinical forms of the disease.

The presence of symptoms was reported by half of the patients. 79% of the patients with erosive lichen planus had some disturbing complication compared with 50% and 37% of the patients with atrophic or reticular forms of the disease, respectively. These findings were highly significant.

Of the group, 49% had no symptoms, whereas 38% had moderate to severe pain. Of those with erosive lichen planus, 59% reported moderate or severe pain compared with only onefifth of those with the reticular form of OLP. The association between the form of OLP and symptoms was highly significant.

Most patients had multiple-site involvement, with the buccal mucosa being the most common location in each clinical form.

71 patients were initially treated with either topical or systemic corticosteroids. In 46 (65%) patients improvement was shown with the use of steroids. Of the remaining 25 patients, 17 (68%) reported no response or improvement less than 50%. However, some improvement, although lower than 50%, was noted in 14 patients.

They concluded that there is no definite mode of treatment for a complete and lasting cure. The main consideration is the satisfactory control of the disease. The administration of medications is mainly used to control discomfort or pain. Corticosteroids, which can be administered systemically or topically, are the most effective modalities. Topical administration of corticosteroids is effective in maintaining a level of satisfactory control. It was found that topical corticosteroids controlled the disease, providing the patient with a general satisfactory quality of life in 65% of treated patients. Because of extreme side effects the use of systemic corticosteroids is limited to short-term and to the most complicated lesions. The recommended dosage for controlling severe OLP is between 40mg to 60mg of prednisone daily for a relatively short time for up to 2 weeks, followed by topical applications of corticosteroids in a form of mouth rinses of dexamethasone elixir 0.1mg/ml, 5ml four times daily, or topical applications of 0.1% triamcinolone acetonide ointment, or 0.1% betamethasone ointment after meals and at bedtime, with orabase used as a vehicle. In stubborn and severe cases in which high doses of systemic corticosteroids are mandatory, a combination of lower doses of corticosteroids with other immune suppressive drugs such as imuran (Azathioprine) or Cyclosporine can be considered.

In this study only 13% of the patients were treated with systemic corticostreroids, and 56% of them improved. However, the small number of patients who were treated with the systemic treatment does not allow any profound conclusions for the efficiency of this systemic medication.

Buajeeb W et al (1997) conducted a study, the purpose of which was to compare the efficacy of retinoic acid in an oral base with fluocinolone acetonide in an oral base in the treatment of atrophic and erosive OLP.

Patients with erosive and atrophic OLP attending the Oral Medicine Clinic, Faculty of Dentistry, Mahidol University in Bangkok were asked to participate in the study.

The drugs under study were fluocinolone acetonide in an oral base 0.1% and retinoic acid in an oral base 0.05%.

Patients were alternately given 0.1% fluocinolone acetonide or 0.05% retinoic acid as they presented to the clinic for treatment. Which medication was used was unknown to patient or clinician. The patients were instructed to apply the medication on dried lesions four times a day. The lesions were evaluated after 2 and 4 weeks of treatment.

Results revealed that eighteen patients (1 man and 17 women) received 0.1% fluocinolone acetonide (group

A) and 15 patients (2 men and 13 women) received 0.05% retinoic acid (group B).

The change noted in the patients receiving the topical fluocinolone acetonide was statistically significantly greater than that in the patients receiving the topical retinoic acid (p=0.01).

They concluded that topical application of fluocinolone acetonide in an orabase 0.1% is a safe and effective treatment of atrophic and erosive OLP.

Carrozzo M, Gandolfo S (1999) reviewed the current literature regarding the medical treatment of OLP.

Single case reports or open trials were included if they covered new therapeutic approaches or suggested significant modifications of known treatment modalities. Review papers were limited to those dealing with the topic.

Every paper was critically examined. Because of the great heterogeneity of the respose criteria, many data could not be directly compared; stronger weight was given to therapies that have proven to be effective under placebo-controlled research protocols. Attention was also drawn to potential and effective adverse effects of every drug used.

They concluded that the various medications advocated for the treatment of OLP, several lack conclusive findings from adequately controlled trials. Mainly high potency topical corticosteroids in an adhesive medium appear at present the safest and most efficacious. Adjuvant agents as antimycotics may be useful along with topical steroid treatment. Systemic corticosteroids may be occasionally indicated for severe recalcitrant erosive OLP or for diffuse mucocutaneous involvement. Topically and systemically delivered retinoids combined with topical corticosteroids could improve the efficacy of these agents whereas complete remission is difficult to achieve with retinoids alone and they frequently cause adverse effects.

Hydrocortisone hemisuccinate pellets or in aqueous solution are often of little benefit in OLP, whereas betamethasone valerate aerosol (800μgd^{-1} for 2 months) has been used successfully. Widespread oral lesions may be treated with high potency steroid mouthwashes such as disodium betamethasone phosphate (0.5 mg dissolved in 10ml warm water, 4 times per day).

Carbone M et al (1999) evaluated the efficacy of a combination of topical corticosteroids with topical antimycotic drugs in the therapy, of atrophic-erosive forms of oral lichen planus (OLP).

The study consisted of 60 patients with OLP subdivided into three groups matched for sex and age. The first group (25 patients) and the second group (24 patients) received respectively 0.05% clobetasol propionate ointment or 0.05% fluocinonide ointment in an adhesive medium (4% hydroxymethyl cellulose gel) plus in each case antimycotic treatment consisting of miconazole gel and 0.12% chlorhexidine mouthwashes. The third group (11 patients), placebo group, received only hydroxyethyl cellulose gel and antimycotic treatment as above. All the treatment regimens were carried out for 6 months. Each patient was examined every 2 months during the 6-months period of active treatment and for a further 6 months of follow-up. Objective and subjective clinical progress was scored and compared between the three groups. Plasma cortisol levels were monitored in the patients using the topical corticosteroids.

They reported that all patients treated with clobetasol and 90% of the patients treated with fluocinonide witnessed some improvement, whereas in the placebo group only 20% of patients improved ($P<0.0001$ and $P=0.00029$, respectively). However, when considering complete responses, only clobetasol gave significantly better results than placebo. Clobetasol resolved 75% of the lesions whereas fluocinonide was effective in 25% of cases and placebo in none. Clobetasol achieved better results statistically than did fluocinonide ($P=0.00442$) and placebo ($P=0.00049$) whereas there was no statistical difference among fluocinonide and placebo ($P=0.140$). Similar results were obtained for symptoms. Both drugs were shown to be effective in the treatment of erosive lesion but clobetasol was considerably more efficacious the fluocinonide in the atrophic areas (75% vs 25% of total response, respectively) ($P=0.00442$). None of the treatment patients contracted oropharyngeal candidiasis. After months of follow-up, 65% of the clobetasol-treated group and 55% of the fluocinonide group were stable. Examination of plasma cortisol levels showed no significant systemic adverse effects of clobetasol or fluocinonide.

They concluded that a very potent topical corticosteroid such as clobetasol may control OLP in most cases, with no significant adrenal suppression or adverse effects. Moreover, a concommitant antimycotic treatment with miconazole gel or chlorhexidine mouthwash is a useful and safe prophylaxis against oropharyngeal candidiasis.

Chainani-WU N et al (2001) describe retrospective, descriptive study using information from patient records at a tertiary referral center. The study included 229 patients with OLP who were seen in the oral medicine clinic at the University of California, San Francisco, between September 1996 and august 2000, for the first time or for a follow-up visit. Signs and symptoms at various clinic visits were quantified. Responses to treatment and disease progression were determined by comparing scores with baseline scores.

The most predictably beneficial medication had been topical corticosteroids, systemic corticosteroids or both because of their profound anti-inflammatory properties. For topical applications, potent corticosteroid forms, which included 0.05 percent fluocinonide gel (Lidex, Medicis), 0.05% fluocinonide oitment mixed with equal parts Orabase paste (Colgate-Palmolive Co.), 0.05% clobetasol gel (Tenovate, GlaxoSmithKline) or 0.05% clobetasol ointment mixed with equal parts Orabase paste was used. Patients were instructed to apply these medications to the lesions one to four times daily.

Prednisone was the systemic corticosteroid used, which was administered in one or two doses a day, for a total daily dosage ranging from 40 to 50 milligrams. In refractive cases or those that were extremely severe, prednisone with the immunosuppressive drug azathioprine (Imuran, FARO pharmaceuticals) in dosages of 50 or 100mg per day was combined. Patients were alerted to the potential adverse side effects of these medications, and their physicians were contacted regarding our diagnosis and suggested treatment; they also were asked if they concurred.

The mean age at onset of the disease was 55 years, and 154 (67%) of the patients were female. Symptoms generally correlated directly with the severity of OLP forms, which ranged from reticular to erosive. Corticosteroids were effective in reducing symptoms, healing ulcers and reducing erythema. At last follow-up, 65% of the patients had the same type of OLP seen initially or the disease had progressed to a more severe type, while 35% of patients had less-severe forms than that seen at the initial visit. Four patients (1.7%) developed oral squamous-cell carcinoma during the follow-up period.

Patients with OLP should be treated if symptoms are significant. Follow-up including supervision of medication use and monitoring of side effects, as well as periodic examinations for possible malignant transformation- is necessary.

ORAL SUBMUCOUS FIBROSIS :

Oral submucous fibrosis (OSMF), a disease due to an insidious, chronic change in fibroelasticity, is characterized by a burning sensation in the oral cavity, blanching and stiffening of the oral mucosa and oropharynx, and trismus. The symptoms and signs depend on the progression of the lesions and on the number of affected sites. More than one oral site is involved in most cases. In advanced lesion, the fibrosis extends from the subepithelial lamina propria through the entire submucosa to the muscle layer. Thick inextensile vertical fibrous bands appear in the cheeks, faucial pillars, and encircle the lips. Narrowing of the oral aperture caused by circular fibrous bands in the lips is not only disfiguring, but also limits oral access, leading eventually to malnutrition and poor oral hygiene. It is considered to be a premalignant stage of oral cancer, affecting predominantly Indians and other Asians.

Sinha and Jain (1978) had tried local injection of hydrocortisone 1.5cc for one group and 2.0cc of Placentrex once a week for the other group for 12 consequent weeks. They reported failure rate 7.2% for hydrocortisone and 31.3% for placentrex and concluded hydrocortisone was superior.

Kakar, Puri et al (1985) recommended four different regimens.

i) 4mg dexamethasone bi weekly

ii) 1500 IU of Hyaluronidase with 1cc of Lignocaine bi weekly

iii) 4mg dexamethasone and 1500 IU of hyaluronidase

iv) 2cc of placental extract bi weekly.

They concluded that No. 3 combination locally for seven weeks could give maximum improvement if it is followed by three weeks of hyaluronidase.

Gupta D, Sharma SC. (1988) conducted a study on a new treatment regimen for oral submucous fibrosis using local injections consisting of a combination of dexamethasone, hyaluronidase and chymotrypsin biweekly for 10 days. Good results were obtained in patients with severe limitation of opening and fibrotic bands with 74% had relief of painful ulceration, 100% relief of burning sensation, 79.5% blanching of oral mucosa and 94% relief of limited opening. Dexamethasone 4mg when used alone had 50% relief of painful ulceration, 82% burning sensation, 56% blanching of oral mucosa and 72% relief of limited opening.

Lai DR et al (1995) reported the treatment of 150 patients divided into two groups with varying degrees of oral submucous fibrosis (OSMF) over a 10-year period (1982-1991), treated by either medical or surgical therapies. Medical treatment involved a) conservative oral administration of vitamin B-complex, buflomedial hydrochloride and topical triamcinolone acetonide 0.1%, or b) conventional submucosal injections of a combination of dexamethasone and hyaluronidase, or c) a combination of both (a) and (b). The surgical group was treated by the excision of fibrotic tissues and covering the defect with split-thickness skin, fresh human amnion, or buccal fat pad (BFP) grafts. Treatment was chosen according to the stage of clinical progression to gain maximal interincisal distance (ID). The cases were followed up by monthly examinations for at least two years, or when possible even longer. A combination of (a) and (b) medical treatment was satisfactory in cases of mild impairment (ID > 20mm) but in the long term it led to symptomatic relief only. Surgical therapy, on the other hand, when accepted by the patients, led to a significant improvement of trismus in cases of severe limitation (ID < 20mm). Following this strategy, an additional ID increase was observed in all patients. BFP grafting was particularly successful in diminishing scarring after two years as compared with the other two grafts. Together with a cessation of the betel quid chewing habit before and after therapy, these treatment regimens combined with daily mouth opening exercises were found to be necessary to manage OSMF cases in early and advanced stages of progression.

Chen H et al (2004) reported a case of facial candida albicans cellulitis occurring in a patient with oral submucous fibrosis and diabetes mellitus after local corticosteroid injection of 40mg triamcinalone acetonide. The symptoms and signs of oral submucous fibrosis improved markedly but facial candidal cellulitis occurred 2 months after the steroid injection.

APHTHOUS STOMATITIS :

Aphthous stomatitis is the most common recurrent oral mucosal ulcerative disease, yet it remains one of the least understood diseases of the oral cavity. Although the term "aphthae" refers simply to the presence of an otherwise undefined ulcer, the disease aphthous stomatitis may appear as lesions localized to the oral mucosa or as a component of vesiculoulcerative disease involving multiple organ systems. The difficulty in establishing the exact nature of aphthous stomatitis is due in part to the nonspecific histopathologic features of the ulcers and to the lack of any reproducibly identifiable cause, endogenous or exogenous.

Cooke BED (1960)[21] conducted a double blind clinical trial to assess the relative value of tablets containing 2.5mg of hydrocortisone hemisuccinate with a lactose base, and an inert preparation of lactose base alone, to patients suffering from RAS. The trial involved 17 patients, each patient was given four tablets a day when the ulcer was present and 2 tablets a day when they were not. Patients were asked to dissolve the tablets in the region of the ulceration. Each patient was given a specially designed form on which they kept record of the duration, site and relative size of the each ulcer. The trial period was for 8 weeks, with an interval period of 2 weeks without treatment. If during the first half of the trial patients were using tablets A, then they had tablets B during second half and viceversa. There was much better clinical response to the drug than to the inert tablet, the difference being greater when the placebo was taken first. During treatment by the drug there was reduction of about 50% in the number of ulcer days and in the number of new ulcers compared with placebo. These differences were highly significant. No side effects were noted by this treatment. The authors concluded that 2.5mg hydrocortisone hemisuccinate given four times daily are of value in reducing by half the degree of ulceration, especially during acute exacerbations.

Macphee IT et al (1968) conducted a double blind pilot study to investigate the effects of triamcinolone acetonide (in orabase) and hydroxyquinolone on a group of 17 patients with RAS with severe continuous ulcer. Orabase (an ointment containing carboxymethylcellulose), was used as a control. Lactose pellets were made up in a form identical with hydroxyquinolone tablets. The order of administration was randomized and the drugs were taken in direct sequence during for 28 days consecutively with no intervening control period. Patients were supplied with a diary in which they recorded the incidence and duration of each ulcer during the entire study period. The dosage of drugs employed were triamcinolone applied 4 times a day (0.24-1mg/day), orabase to be applied 4 times daily and one 0.65mg tablet of hydroxyquinolone swallowed 3 times a day whether the lesions were present or not. The groups were compared for the number of new ulcers for 28 days and the mean duration of ulcers, the differences were not statistically significant. The authors concluded that triamcinolone given over a period of 4 weeks in the dose range used was unlikely to be effective against aphthous ulcers of the degree of severity selected for the trial.

Pimlott SJ and Walker DM (1983) conducted a randomized single blind crossover trial to evaluate the efficacy of 0.05% fluocinonide in orabase in treatment of RAS and also tested for any adrenal suppression as a result of treatment in 22 patients with RAS. The medication was to be applied 5-6 times daily for six weeks. After a interval period of 2 weeks of no therapy, the alternative preparation was prescribed for a further 6 weeks. The patients were also asked to make a daily assessment of pain or discomfort on a VAS, and to enter the number of ulcers, any new lesions and the number of times the preparation was used. The mean number of new ulcers, mean number of ulcer days, mean number of ulcer free days, average pain score during ulcer days and average duration of ulcers in days were compared between active and the placebo group. Short tetracosactrin tests were performed before and after the trial to monitor adrenal function. 20 of the 22 patients completed the trial. 18 of these 20 patients preferred active preparation where as the other 2 had no preference. There was no significant differences between the mean number of new ulcers and average pain score, however there was a significant reduction in the number of mean number of ulcer days and average duration of ulcers and an increase in the number of ulcer free days. The corticosteroid also did not suppress adrenal gland function. The authors found the results of the study encouraging, and stressed on the need for a longer trial period to monitor long-term control of oral ulceration.

Miles DA et al (1993) conducted a randomized control trial on 30 RAS patients for 12 weeks to compare the efficacy of 0.025% triaminolone acetonide and 0.12% chlorhexidine gluconate solution, placed under a physical barrier of cyanoacrylate. Group I received triamcinolone, group 2 0.12% chlorhexidine and group 3 cyanoacrylate only. Patients were instructed to keep a diary to record their pain level on a 10cm VAS until the lesion healed. 19 patients completed the study. The results revealed highly significant differences in pain intensity between the 3 test groups. There was no difference found between the groups with respect to the duration of the lesion. They concluded that there was no noticeable reduction in the total number of ulcer days with either chlorhexidine or triamcinolone. However, there was a significant reduction in pain intensity almost immediately after application of either of these agents and both agents improved the symptoms better than physical barrier alone.

Rhodus NL and Berenter Janna (1998) conducted a clinical trial to compare triamcinalone acetonide 0.1% in orabase with a chemical cautery agent, consisting of 50% sulfuric acid and 28% sulfonated phenolics in aqueous solution in treatment of RAS patients. The rationale for use of this chemical cautery agent is that it cauterizes the epithelial tissue affected by the immune response. Sixty patients with RAS were enrolled. 20 patients were assigned to each treatment group. 20 age and sex matched patients were enrolled in the control group and these patients received no treatment. Clinical assessments of all subjects were made at days 0, 3, 6 and 10. The maximum diameter of the ulcer and the erythematous halo was recorded at each visit. Subjective evaluations of subjects symptoms were made by subjects perception of pain from the ulcer on a 100mm VAS scale. The test agents were applied topically to the lesions. The chemical cautery agent was applied to the ulcers, a single time, directly over the margins of the ulccr for a pcriod of 10 scconds. Thc arca was then thoroughly flushed with water and dried thoroughly with cotton application. Triamcinolone was applied liberally over the ulcer 3 times daily by the subject.

Following treatment the size of the ulcer had not changed significantly in any of the groups by day 3. However a significant decrease in VAS in the patients receiving chemical cautery agent indicated a significant improvement in pain (>70%) as compared to the triamcinolone groups (<20%) and ocntrol group (>30%). By day 6, 7% of the ulcers had clinically disappeared, and there was resolution of symptoms in 100% of the subjects in the cautery agent group. Only 30% lesions disappeared in the other groups. By day 10, 100% of the ulcers had clinically healed and were causing no pain in both treatment groups at day 10, 10% of the control group still had clinical ulcers present, with an average VAS of 18mm. The results indicated that immediate and significant relief of the pain accompanying RAS was achieved in patients on chemical cautery agent treatment. The clinical healing was also better in this group. They concluded that relief of the symptoms in RAS patients may or maynot correspond to clinical improvement and these 2 medications may affect signs and symptoms of RAS differently.

Muzio LL et al (2001) evaluated the effects of topical corticosteroid therapy in association with agents that increased the adhesion of the active drug to the oral mucosa in 30 RAS patients. The first group received 0.05% clobetasol propionate, second group applied the drug in an adhesive denture paste while third group applied the drug in an oral analgesic paste. Each patient was examined on the days when symptoms were present. They observed that the drug reduced the healing time in most patients and more significantly in the groups treated with adhesive denture paste. They concluded that the use of clobetasol propionate in association with a denture adhesive had greater level of effectiveness as compared to the use of medication alone or with benzocaine containing orabase.

PEMPHIGUS VULGARIS :

Lozada F, Silverman S, Cram D (1982) conducted a clinical trial to assess the benefits and clinical efficacy of combination of prednisone and levamisole in the treatment of PV.

Six patients with mucocutaneous PV diagnoses were confirmed by clinical findings and tissue evaluation using routine staining and immuno-fluorescence techniques. All six were selected for this study because of the high minimum effective dose of prednisone required for long-term control (40 to 80 mg. daily). All of these patients already had developed corticosteroid side effects.

Levamisole was chosen to supplement and, it was hoped, reduce the prednisone regimens as well as to enhance disease control. All prednisone doses were lowered below those previously required to control signs and symptoms. Levamisole was arbitrarily administered as 50 mg. every other day in four patients and 150 mg. a day for 3 days each week in two patients. Both prednisone and levamisole dosages were adjusted during the course of treatment, depending upon clinical responses and occurrences of side effects. The object was to assess the lowest combination dosage that would satisfactorily control signs and symptoms.

All patients responded within 2 to 8 weeks. The minimum effective dose range of prednisone when used with levamisole was reduced to 5 to 35 mg. daily. A temporary minor side effect occurred in only one patient. This corticosteroid-sparing, combination-drug approach for patients with PV has resulted in acceptable clinical control and diminution of the side effects that often interfere with high-dosage, long-term treatment.

Paterson AJ, Lamey PJ, Lewis Nolan A, Rademaker M (1993) reported a case of a 78-year-old patient complaining of oral ulceration which had been present for seven days. Intra-oral examination revealed mucosal sloughing of the hard and soft palate, both lateral borders of the tongue, floor of mouth and labial aspect of the lower lip. Extra-oral examination revealed a bullous lesion on the skin of the lower trunk.

The patient was known to have asthma, which had been well controlled for approximately 5 years by beclomethasone inhaler (100 μg, 8-hourly), salbutamol inhaler (as required) and aminophylline (225 mg, 12-hourly). In addition he had been diagnosed as having maturity-onset diabetes mellitus three years previously and this had been controlled by diet alone. However, fourteen days prior to presentation the patient had been put on glibenclamide therapy (5 mg, 12-hourly).

Indirect immunofluorescence was positive at a titre of 1 /160 to intercellular IgG and C3. Direct immunofluorescence was positive for intercellular IgG and C3, which was reported as being consistent with pemphigus vulgaris. The patient was instructed to stop glibenclamide and put on 40 mg prednisolone daily. At review after a further 5 days the patient reported that his oral and cutaneous lesions had resolved within 48 hours of the start of treatment.

The patient was advised to reduce his prednisolone gradually by 5 mg daily. After 2 weeks the patient felt that his lesions might be about to recur and was therefore give azathioprine (100 mg b.d.). During the subsequent 2 weeks one skin lesion developed and therefore the patient was hospitalized. Indirect immunofluorescence showed a circulating pemphigus antibody of 1 / 1280, random venous plasma blood glucose was within normal range and an oral rinse yielded no significant growth. The patient's metformin (850 mg, 12-hourly) therapy was maintained but prednisolone (20 mg daily) reinduced resolution of oral lesions occurred within 48 hours. After a further 48 hours the patient was discharged on 10 mg prednisolone and 100 mg azathioprine daily. At subsequent outpatient review he has remained asymtpomatic for 12 months.

Robinson JC, Lozada-Nur F, Frieden I, Francisco S, Calif. (1997)[77] conducted a study to illustrate the natural course of oral PV disease and to describe the different treatment modalities used.

The study group consisted of 12 patients with oral PV. There were nine women and three men. Diagnoses were established by clinical appearance of the disease and biopsy with hematoxylin and eosin staining. Biopsy with direct immunofluorescence was performed when that procedure was considered necessary and had not been previously performed by the referring health care provider. Thorough medical history and oral examination were performed on all patients by the same clinician. Treatment was undertaken with the goal of achieving complete control of signs and symptoms of the disease, with minimal side effects. They were treated with systemic prednisone and / or topical corticosteroids and an adjunctive systemic medication, which included azathioprine, levamisole, cyclosporine, methotrexate, and dapsone. Topical agents included fluocinonide 0.05% (Lidex), clobetasol 0.05% (Tenovate), or halobetasol o.05% (Ultravate) ointments compounded 1:1 with Orabase. Dexamethasone elixir, 0.1 mg / ml, was used topically by having the patient hold 5 ml (1 teaspoonful) in the mouth for 4 to 5 minutes and then expectorate; this was to be done preferably after meals and at bedtime. For lesions that were primarily gingival, fluocinonide gel was used in custom-made applicator trays, which were vaccum-formed soft plastic trays relieved around the gingivae and with borders that extended almost to the vestibular sulcus. Applicator trays were used only for maintenance therapy, not for initial induction therapy, to prevent further tearing of gingival tissues. At each clinic visit, patients were monitored for signs of Candida albicans by clinical appearance, potassium hydroxide staining, or culture. Throughout the course of therapy, patients received some form of antifungal therapy, either topically (nystatin vaginal suppositories used as oral lozenges) or systemically (Ketaconazole or fluconazole) as initial therapy or as secondary prophylaxis. The initial dose of prednisone was maintained for 2 to 3 weeks, especially in patients with initial severe disease. The endpoint of the initial treatment was considered to have been reached when the patient was asymptomatic and control of clinical signs was observed. In one case, initial therapy consisted only of the use of topical corticosteroids. The other 11 patients were treated with 2 to 6 weeks of high to moderate dose prednisone with or without initial adjunctive therapy. In all cases, dosages were tapered, as disease response would allow. 11 patients experienced side effects as a result of the prolonged therapy required for disease control. Nine patients eventually experienced complete remission. The others achieved a significant reduction in disease severity and frequency of disease exacerbations, or "flares," during maintenance-phase therapy. One patient was not able to take therapeutic doses of prednisone because she developed severe psychosis, limiting her management and disease control.

Our series demonstrates he value of early diagnosis and the effect of early treatment on prognosis and the course of disease. In fact, long-term follow-up information on this group of patients, although small, suggests that, with time and low-dose combination therapy regimens, PV eventually tends to quiet down, as illustrated by less severe and frequent flare-ups.

Sirois D. Janet E. Leigh Thomas P. Sollecito (2000) described the clinical presentation of 42 cases of oral PV evaluated and diagnosed by dentists Emphasis is placed on the distribution and appearance of oral PV lesions and diagnosis of the disease.

Systemic corticosteroids are the first line of therapy of treatment of PV. When prednisone was introduced for the treatment of PV, doses often were excessive (more than 200 milligrams per day) and were associated with considerable morbidity. Lower doses (0.5 to 1 mg per kilogram of body weight) proved to be very effective and associated with less morbidity. Nonetheless, prednisone should be prescribed only by clinicians who have experience in monitoring and managing steroid-related complications. Most patients with PV receive a second immunosuppressant drug to achieve a complete remission. The most common drug combination is prednisone with either azathioprine or cyclophosphamide. These drugs not only provide additional immunoregulatory benefit, leading to complete remission, but also have steroid-sparing properties that allow the dose of prednisone to be reduced significantly. More recently, mycophenolate mofetil has been shown to allow significant prednisone dose reduction and complete remission with fewer side effects.

Several approaches are available to minimize the side effects of long-term corticosteroid use, including alternate-day dosing and combination therapy with steroid-sparing medications. Systemic corticosteroids should be prescribed only by clinicians trained in and familiar with their use. The most important aspect of PV is its early recognition, diagnosis and a unique opportunity to make the diagnosis and then refer the patient to a dental or medical specialists for treatment.

Mignogna MD, Muzio LL, Mignogna RE et al (2000) studied 16 patient with pemphigus vulgaris (11 women and 5 men) with age between 26 to 76 yr. All the patient complained of symptoms such as oral pain, dysphagia and odyno phagia because of the extensive mucosal erosion.

The protocol for the initial / induction phase of treatment consisted of systemic deflazacort (120 mg daily in a single morning dose) and topical corticosteroids. The initial dose of deflazacort was maintained from 2-4 weeks especially in patients with severe initial disease. In addition, in the case of PV unresponsive to the conventional high dose of steroids, patients received adjunctive systemic mediation, which included azathioprine (50 to 100 mg daily) or cyclophosphamide (50 mg daily). In two cases "pulse therapy with methylprednisolone" (1 grain methylprednisolone daily for 3 days repeated after 21 days) was performed.

Topical agents included 0.05% clobetasol (Clobesol) ointment mixed 1:1 with orabase. For lesions that were primarily gingival, clobetasol was used in custom-made applicator trays that were made of vacuum-formed soft plastic relieved around the gingivae and with borders that extended almost to the vestibular reflex.

Following clinical remission, the patients' dosage of deflazacort was tapered to 6 mg every other day. During this period calcium and vitamin D were usually administered as dietary supplements.

Fourteen patients received systemic deflazacort at a dose of 120 mg (100 mg of prednisone equivalent) daily. The initial dose was maintained from 2 to 4 weeks until remission; remission was determined as a state in which approximately 75% of the old lesions were healed and no new lesions developed. At the fourth week, patients 4,5,7,8,11 and 15 showed incomplete or no remission, so we started the adjunctive therapy with azathioprine (50 mg/bid): remission occurred in all cases after 2 to 4 weeks. In all cases deflazacort dosages were tapered as disease response would allow. Azathioprine was gradually tapered only when the deflazacort dosage was less than 45 mg every other day without relapse. In seven cases we had one or more relapses during maintenance-phase therapy: a relapse was defined as the appearance of more than five new lesions within a period of 3 days; smears, biopsy specimens. DIF and IIF investigations were always performed after a relapse. Relapses were treated by doubling the steroid dose administered at the time.

The most common adverse events during treatment were insomnia and mood alterations. In case 2, there was an acute psychosis during the steroid tapering phase; it responded well to antipsychotic drugs. We constantly observed a moderate increase of white blood cells, and of platelets in two cases.

Allen CM, Camisa C (2000) stated that management of PV with a variety of immunosuppressive regimens has been attempted, but the degree of success is somewhat limited. While high-dose systemic corticosteroid therapy (1-2 mg of oral prednisone/kg daily) remains the mainstay of treatment, other immune-modulating agents have been combined with prednisone in hopes of improving survival, although dramatic improvement in survival rates has not generally been seen (Anhalt, 1997). These agents include azathioprine (Camisa et al, 1992), methotrexate, cyclophosphamide (Perniciaro et al, 1994; lemon et al, 1997) gold salts, dapsone, plasmapheresis (lemon et al, 1997) and photopheresis. Pulse therapy using cyclophosphamide combined with dexamethasone has also been reported to have a favourable impact on the disease process (Backer et al, 1998). For those patients whose PV is associated with chronic lymphocytic leukemia (CLL), a better response seems to have been documented when systemic corticosteroids were combined with cyclosporine (5 mg kg daily).

Muhammad KJ. Lewis MAO. Crean SJ. (2002) a 28-year-old Caucasian female presented at the oral medicine clinic on an emergency basis with a five-week history of oro-pharyngeal ulceration, which was becoming increasingly painful and more widespread. The case records revealed that the patient had been seen eight months earlier complaining of pain from her gingivae and palate. A routine mucosal biopsy demonstrated histopatholgoical features that were suggestive of either Erythema multiforme or pemphigus vulgaris. A clinical diagnosis of Erythema multiforme had been preferred due to short duration of symptoms and the young age of the patient. This clinical diagnosis was supported by the total resolution of the original symptoms following a short course of systemic steroids.

At the time of eventual re-presentation the patient indicated that she was 12 weeks pregnant and the ulceration had started 8 weeks into the pregnancy. The pain associated with the oral symptoms was limiting her ability to eat and she was becoming increasingly worried that poor intake of food was going to harm the development of the foetus.

Extra-oral clinical examination was unremarkable. Intra-oral examination revealed extensive areas of erosion affecting the upper labial mucosa, soft palate, floor of the mouth, gingivae and buccal mucosa. The level of oral hygiene was poor and there was marked halitosis. A provisional diagnosis of a vesiculo-bullous condition was made, with a differential diagnosis of Erythema multiforme, mucous membrane pemphigoid and pemphigus vulgaris. There was no improvement in the symptoms despite treatment with topical betamethasone, 0.5 mg tablet dissolved in water and used as a mouth-wash for two minutes, three times daily. In addition, the patient was provided with a beclomethasone inhaler and instructed to direct two puffs (250μg each) at the affected mucosa twice daily, if symptoms failed to improve. At review after a further five days, the lesions were failing to resolve and a diagnosis of Erythema multiforme was now thought unlikely.

Histopathological examination of a haematoxylin and eosin stained preparation showed suprabasal clefting and acantholysis, features consistent with PV. Direct immunofluorescence on fresh tissue was positive and revealed the presence of IgG in the intercellular spaces throughout the epithelium, a pattern of immunofluorescence consistent with a diagnosis of PV. Patient required systemic steroid therapy. Further management of the patient was discussed with her obstetrician, before a decision was made to prescribe prednisolone 20 mg orally once per day. At review one week later, the oral lesions had improved considerably and the pain reduction had enabled the patient to return to a normal diet. Over the next three weeks, the dose of prednisolone was gradually reduced by 5 mg increments per week and brought to a level of 5 mg once a day. This low level of prednisolone was continued for the duration of the pregnancy without any recurrence of the oral lesions. The pregnancy and the delivery were uneventful and a healthy boy, weighing 10 lb 2oz, was delivered at term by caesarean section under epidural anaesthesia and appropriate steroid cover.

BELL'S PALSY :

Idiopathic (Bell's) facial palsy is a self-limiting non-fatal and spontaneously remitting disorder of acute onset due to non-suppurative inflammation of the facial nerve within the stylomastoid foramen.

Muralidhar M et al (1987) reviewed the treatment of Bell's palsy and stated that one of the oldest attempts was the use of cortisone as advocated by Robinson and

Moss in 1954. Taverner and cowroerks found that ACTH was more effective if given early. In subsequent studies, the same authors found that prednisone 40 mg qid for 5days followed by diminishing doses proved superior to the ACTH therapy. Adour began using orally administered prednisone in treating Bell's palsy in 1970 after demonstrating poor results on surgical decompression of the facial nerve. He began the treatment with 40mg prednisone daily for 4 days and tapered to 8mg daily in 8 days. In a continuation of the same study, Adour attempted a change of therapeutic regime. One mg prednisone was given per kg per day for 10-15 days which he believed to give better results. Hall and Colman also advocated predisone therapy (80mg in divided doses for 5 days and tapered for the next 5 days).

Papazian MR, Campbell JA and Nabi S (1993) stated that if the patient is seen within 2 to 3 weeks of onset of symptoms, prednisone in doses of 1mg/kg/d for 10 to 14 days has been recommended, as long as there are no medical contraindications.

Proposed guidelines for steroid usage in Bell's palsy

Presentation within 3 weeks of onset

Prednisone 1mg/kg/d, with a gradual taper

Example dosage for a 60-kg female

Prednisone, 10mg tablets : 3 oral twice-daily doses for 4 days then 2 oral twice daily doses for 4 days then 1 oral twice daily dose for 4 days, then 1 oral daily dose for 4 days then stop

The hope is that the steroids might speed the recovery time and prevent synkinesis.

Ko JY et al (2000) treated thirty patients suffering from facial palsy secondary to herpes zoster infection of the auriculo-temporal region. Combination of parenteral acyclovir and oral prednisolone showed dramatic relief in most cases. Age and multiple nerve involvements were major negative prognosticating factors.

MUCOCELE :

Mucocele is a term used to describe swellings caused by the pooling of saliva at the site of an injured minor salivary gland duct. The majority of these lesions occur on the lower lip. Mucoceles may be divided into a mucus extravasation type and a mucus retention type. The mucus extravasation type is the common mucocele and is caused by the laceration of a minor salivary gland duct by trauma. Saliva leaks into the submucosal tissues causing pooling of mucus, resulting in inflammation and formation of granulation tissue.

Tulio M (1976) reported that mucoceles may be treated by injection of a steroid preparations. Although the author claimed success in only three of eight cases, the simplicity of the treatment indicates that it should be tried before resorting to surgery.

Wilcox JW, Hickory JE (1979) treated 14 cases of mucocele of the lip. Small syringe with a half-inch, 26-gauge needle was used to inject triamcinolone acetate. No anesthetic was required. A steady injection is applied until the overlying mucosa is thoroughly distended. The average lesion requires from 0.5 to 1.5 ml. Results showed that the patients had not complained about discomfort from the injection other than the sensation of enlargement of the lip. After a single injection in 12 of the 14 cases, there were no recurrence for periods of observation of 16 to 24 months.

One patient, who was seen on two occasions, was referred for treatment of multiple mucoceles after a vermilionectomy. When he received the second injection, he had an immediate mild systemic allergic reaction to the medication. This reaction was resolved by administration of 50 mg Benadryl intramuscularly. Fortunately, a third treatment was not necessary. There was only one case of mucocele that required a series of four injections.

They concluded that mechanism of action of the steroid is unclear apparently the injected steroid either causes pressure atrophy of the feeding gland or resolution of the associated inflammation, or both.

PSORIASIS :

Psoriasis is a relatively common chronic dermatological disease characterized by epithelial hyperplasia presenting clinically as cutaneous erythematous papules and plaques covered by whitish scales commonly observed on the extensor-dorsal cutaneous surfaces. Although the etiology of psoriasis remains unclear, the epithelial changes are related to a defect in the control of keratiocyte proliferation. Most agree that intraoral psoriasis usually occurs in the presence of cutaneous disease.

Younai FS and Phelan JA (1997) reported a case of a 65-year-old Russian woman who presented to the clinical oral pathology service for evaluation of a lesion on her upper lip that had been present for 4 years. Her medical history was significant for peripheral vascular disease and hypertension. Medications prescribed by her physician included reserpine and two topical ointments, fluocinonide and acyclovir, which she occasionally used for the lip lesion. Clinical examination revealed a 1x3 cm lesion on the upper lip that exhibited a crusted surface. The crust was loosely adherent, and removal revealed tiny areas of bleeding and pinpoint white specks that appeared pustular and could not be rubbed off. The mucosa under her maxillary partial denture was erythematous and exhibited a granular texture similar to that seen in denture associated stomatitis. The tongue was fissured with areas resembling geographic tongue, and lesions resembling ectopic geographic tongue were present on the buccal mucosa, lower lip, and floor of the mouth. The entire buccal and labial mucosa, the involved portion of the hard palate, and the tongue exhibited multiple pustules that could not be rubbed off. Examination of the exposed skin, scalp, and nails revealed no cutaneous lesions. The patient denied the presence or a history of any associated skin lesions in the perianal or genital regions.

Biopsy of the lesion of the lip and lesions of the hard palate were performed, which revealed lack of fungal hypae on either superficial smear or in tissue sections which were suggestive of a diagnosis of psoriasis.

On the basis of the bacterial culture and antibiotic sensitivity tests, the patient was given erythromycin 250 mg four times daily for 5 days. Topical fluocinonide (Lidex) 0.05% ointment mixed in equal parts with Orbase was also prescribed, to be applied four times a day to the lip and oral mucosa including the denture-bearing area.

Examination after 5 days showed complete resolution of all lesions. The lip lesions healed with slight pigmentation remaining in the area, and no evidence of pustules was present either on the lip or intraorally.

Brice DM, Danesh-Meyer MJ (2000) reported the case of a 51 year-old male with persistent redness on his gingiva. The patients medical history revealed that he was not presently taking any medications and had no known allergies. He reported being diagnosed with psoriasis by a dermatologist approximately 5 years previously, following the appearance of cutaneous lesions on his forearms and legs. The lesions appeared as small erythematous papules and plaque like areas covered with fine whitish-silvery scales. The lesions resolved spontaneously after a period of approximately 12 months and the patient reported no further cutaneous lesions. This remission of cutaneous lesions persisted even after the patient presented with oral lesions.

The patient reported with the appearance of reddish/whitish lesions on his attached gingiva, which had been present for approximately 6 months and bled occasionally on brushing. The patient had received a full-mouth scaling from his general dentist 3 months previously, which failed to resolve the problem, and he was subsequently referred for further investigation.

A full thickness incisional biopsy of the gingiva, including the free gingival margin and attached gingiva was performed which was suggestive of intraoral psoriasis. The patient received further scaling, prophylaxis, and careful oral hygiene instruction. In addition the patient was prescribed a corticosteroid mouthwash, betamethasone (three or four 0.5mg tablets dissolved in glass of warm water) and rinsed twice daily for 2 to 3 weeks. The patient was brought back for a further reevaluation at 6 weeks. Clinically, there was a significant improvement in the patients gingival condition. There was very little erythema remaining around the gingival margins and no bleeding on probing and the patient remarked that his mouth generally felt more comfortable. The patient was placed on a 3 month maintenance programme. At 12 months, the patients gingival condition remained stable, with no clinically detectable intraoral lesions.

ERYTHEMA MULTIFORME :

Erythema multiforme (EM) is a chronic inflammatory mucocutaneous disease that can occur in both genders at any age. Although the cause remains obscure, a wide range of antigens and factors – including herpesvirus and bacterial infections, radiation therapy, and malignancy – have been suggested as triggering the disease.

Lozada F (1981) conducted an open clinical trial to assess the synergistic effect of azathioprine with prednisone, comparing clinical benefits with side effects. Twelve patients were studied. The minimum effective dose of prednisone when used alone was 40mg daily, whereas the minimum effective dose of prednisone when used with azathioprine was never more than 25mg daily and ranged as low as 5mg daily. This study indicated that azthioprine effectively reduced corticosteroid requirement, allowing lower doses of prednisone with satisfactory clinical efficacy and a marked reduction in side effects.

Konstantinidis AB, Markopoulos A, Trigonides G (1985) reported a case of 37 year-old white man who was referred to the department of oral medicine, dental school, university of Thessaloniki, Greece, with a complaint of "sore mouth" of about one week's duration. He mentioned a history of recurrent intraoral painful vesicles and ulcerations accompanied by a low-grade fever in April 1962, Feb. 1966, May 1980 and the last one in May 1982 for which he was referred to us. All the signs and symptoms appeared after oral administration of ampicillin given for another reason.

Ten days prior to the onset of symptoms the patient began taking ampicillin 250 mg, four times daily, on the advice of his physician for the treatment of a gram negative bacterial infection. He continued to take the drug until one day before the oral symptoms began. The lesion from the lip was biopsied. From the histological and clinical features a diagnosis of EM was established. The patient was given betamethasone phosphate tables 0.5mg four times daily. After six days the dosage was decreased, and within two weeks therapy with betamethasone phosphate had been discontinued. He showed prompt improvement and a final elimination of the symptoms during the short course of therapy.

Cohen DM, Bhattacharyya I (2000) reported a case of a 66-year-old woman with a chief complaint of soreness associated with large ulcers that had been present in her mouth continuously for the past four months.

On examination large areas of serpiginous ulcerations on the labial and buccal mucosa and on the ventral surface of the tongue, and swollen lips were seen. A biopsy of the buccal mucosa at the first appointment was done.

Patient was placed on a regimen of 40mg of prednisone (in tablet form) daily for five days, dose was then reduced gradually over the next two weeks. She returned after one week, and dramatic improvement in her condition was noted. The erosions and ulcers in her mouth had healed completely. When the patient returned two weeks later, she had recurrent punctate ulcers on the left anterior buccal mucosa and hard palate. The area where the biopsy was performed appeared red and irritated. At this time, the patient was given a regimen of topical fluocinonide 0.05 percent gel.

Multiple ulcers all over her mouth were present for the past six months. She had been prescribed prednisone tablets by her physician, which helped to a small extent. She also had intermittent smaller lesions, which she had self-medicated with topical fluocinonide 0.05 percent gel. At this appointment, they found diffuse red areas with small ulcers on the anterior mucosal aspect of the upper lip and on the left buccal mucosa. They also observed a small ulcer on the ventral surface of the tongue. During that appointment, she reported consuming cinnamon-flavored bread pudding immediately before the onset of the latest outbreak and confessed to frequently using cinnamon-flavored sugar on bread and rolls, as well as drinking herbal tea with cinnamon daily.

She was advised to avoid cinnamon completely and once again prescribed 40mg of prednisone tablets daily. She returned approximately one week later and the lesions were almost completely healed except for some residual soreness. Again topical fluocinonide 0.05% gel was prescribed. The patient was seen again after two weeks, and there was complete resolution of all the symptoms with no evidence of any lesions.

HERPES VIRUS INFECTIONS :

VZV causes two distinct infections, a primary infection, varicella (chickenpox), and a recurrent infection, herpes zoster (shingles).

After primary infection, VZV becomes latent in dorsal root or cranial nerve ganglia. In 0.3% to 0.5% of the population, the virus becomes reactivated, causing herpes zoster. The nerves most commonly affected with herpes zoster are C-3, T-5, L-1 and L-2. When herpes zoster involves the trigeminal ganglion, the first division (ophthalmic) is most commonly involved, and eye involvement becomes a potentially serious complication. Consultation with an ophthalmologist is necessary in these cases.

A potential sequela of herpes zoster is post herpetic neuralgia (PHN) resulting from scarring of the involved nerve during infection. PHN is a painful, sometimes debilitating condition that can last from months to years after the lesions are healed. The incidence of PHN is increased in patients over 50, and some investigators report that use of a short course of systemic corticosteroids decreases the incidence of PHN, but the usefulness of this recommendation is disputed. Corticosteroid therapy has been used in the hope that it might decrease the neural inflammation and associated chronic pain.

Whitley RJ, Weiss H et al (1996) conducted randomized and controlled studies on 208 immunocompetent patients above the age of 50. A total of 15 university hospitals were enrolled for the study. They preferred following doses : acyclovir 800 mg 5 times a day for 21 days and prednisone for 21 days on 60 mg per day for first 7 days, 30mg / day for next 7 days, and 15 mg/day for last 7 days. Suitable matched placebo were also included in the study. Combined acyclovir and prednisone therapy can improve quality of life in older age group patients who are immunocompetent was the recommendation of this group.

Ernst ME et al (1998) have warned against indiscriminate use of corticosteroids for prevention of PHN. They mentioned that although systemic dissemination of virus is a possibility in clinics it is rarely actually encountered. The older patients chosen for this therapy must be healthy in all other respects with no trace of immunocompromise.

RAMSAY HUNT SYNDROME :

The strict definition of the Ramsay Hunt syndrome is peripheral facial nerve palsy accompanied by an erythematous vesicular rash on the ear (zoster oticus) and in the mouth. J Ramsay Hunt, who described various clinical presentations of facial paralysis and rash, also recognized other frequent symptoms and signs such as tinnitus, hearing loss, nausea, vomitting, vertigo, and nystagmus. He explained these eighth nerve features by the close proximity of the geniculate ganglion to the vestibulocochlear nerve within the bony facial canal. Hunt's analysis of clinical variations of the syndrome now bearing his name led to his recognition of the general somatic sensory function of the facial nerve and his defining of the geniculate zone of the ear. It is now known that varicella zoster virus (VZV) causes Ramsay Hunt syndrome. Compared with Bell's palsy (facial paralysis without rash), patients with Ramsay Hunt syndrome often have more severe paralysis at onset and are less likely to recovery completely.

Sweeney CJ, Gilden DH (2001) suggested that f all patients with Ramsay Hunt syndrome or Bell's palsy with a 7-10 day course of famciclovir (500mg, three times daily) or acyclovir (800mg, five times daily), as well as oral prednisone (60mg daily for 3-5 days). Finally, some patients develop peripheral facial paralysis without ear or mouth rash, associated with either a fourfold rise in antibody to VZV or the presence of VZV DNA in auricular skin, blood mononuclear cells, middle ear fluid, or saliva. This indicates that a proportion of patients with "Bell's palsy" have Ramsay Hunt syndrome zoster sine herpes. Treatment of these patients with acyclovir and prednisone within 7 days of onset has been shown to improve the outcome of recovery from facial palsy.

CENTRAL GIANT CELL GRANULOMA :

The central giant cell granuloma, or CGCG, is a benign intraosseous lesion of the jaw. It is found predominantly in children and young adults. It is an asymptomatic lesion, which often becomes evident on routine radiographic examination. Giant cell lesions have been described as both nonaggressive and aggressive in nature, with recurrence noted in cases of aggressive lesions. Central giant cell lesions present as unilocular or multilocular radiolucent lesions on radiographs. Multinucleated giant cells within a collagenous stroma are the characteristic histopathologic features of CGCG.

Kermer C, Millesi W, Watzke IM (1994) reported a case of 40-year old man referred with a multilocular osteolytic lesion in the right body of the mandible. The patient had partial dentition showing periodontal disease and multiple cavities. The initial therapeutic procedure comprised of adequate periodontal treatment, and a biopsy of the lesion was taken. Histopathologic analysis revealed a CGCG. The laboratory findings revealed no evidence of primary hyperparathyroidism.

Three weeks after the extractions, local injection with corticosteroids was started. The procedure was done as follows: equal parts of triamcinolone acetonide (Volon A® 10 mg) and lidocaine (Xhylanaest® 0.5%) were mixed. Approximately 3 ml of solution was injected into the lesion by multiple penetrations with a needle of 0.5 mm in diameter. Not more than 2ml of solution per 2 cms of radiolucency on the panoramic radiograph should be injected at one time. The injections were done weekly. In week 6, penetration of the cortex overlying the osteolytic zone was no longer feasible ; this determined the end of the treatment. Three weeks after termination of the intralesional injections, bony regeneration could be observed radiologically.

The patient was seen at regular intervals, and 14 months after the initial treatment ended, a solitary bony lesion was diagnosed in the sysmphysis of the mandible, as well as multiple small cystic alterations on the left side of the ramus. After a repeat biopsy and histopathologic confirmation of the diagnosis, local corticosteroids were again applied as described before. Bony consolidation could be observed within weeks. Total follow-up after the first interference was 3 years, and radiographs showed no recurrence and good bony consolidation.

Terry BC, Jacoway JR. (1994) presented an alternative nonsurgical method for managing giant cell lesion in the bone as reported by Dr. Francis V. Howell of LaJolla. The authors also reported 5 cases that were treated using the same protocol as mentioned above and obtained satisfactory results.

Dr. Francies V. Howell of La Jolla, California, conceived an alternative nonsurgical method for managing giant cell lesions in bone. His protocol was as follows

1) Biopsy for histopathological diagnosis.
2) Intralesional injection of a mixture consisting of equal parts of triamcinolone acetonide (10mg/ml) (Kenalog-10) and a local anesthetic (Marcaine 0.5% with epinephrine 1:200,000). The suggested dosage of this mixture was 2 ml per estimated 2cm of radiolucency. (Howell FV: personal communication).

The injections were given on a weekly basis for 6 weeks. It was recommended that a 1- or 2-mm syringe be used with a small-gauge needle (26 guage), to allow the mixture to be forcibly injected ; penetration with a small needle prevents the medication from being expelled through the previous penetration sites on subsequent injections. Although the mixture was injected under considerable pressure, multiple penetrations, especially in large lesions, may be required to be certain that it reaches all areas of the lesion. In some cases, it was noted that after the third week it became more difficult to place the needle into the lesion and a reduced amount of the mixture could injected, indicating a rapid resolution. When the series of injections were completed, the patient showed continued resolution of signs, such as tightening of mobile teeth, reduction in discomfort, and return to normal anatomic contours. Radiographic changes to a more normal bony trabecular pattern could be noted after 3 to 6 months. When there was a positive response without complete resolution, a second series of injections were recommended. Incomplete resolution may represent areas of the lesion that were not reached by the mixture. In the event that there are no clinical or radiographic signs of resolution with this treatment, and if there was continued growth and destruction, immediate surgical intervention was recommended.

They believed that sufficient evidence existed to warrant this nonsurgical mode of therapy as the first choice in the management of giant cell lesion in bone. They also suggested that a long-term, controlled, prospective study of this lesion should be established to provide documentation and verification of the efficacy of this nonsurgical treatment modality.

Adornato MC, Paticoff KA (2001) reported a case of a 10-year-old girl with an expansile lesion of the mandible. The panoramic radiograph showed a well-circumscribed mixed radiolucent-radiopaque lesion of the left mandibular body. An incisional biopsy of the lesion was performed to establish a histologic diagnosis. The specimen was submitted for frozen-section examination, and a diagnosis of CGCG was made. Serum calcium, parathyroid hormone and phosphorous levels were normal.

They administered intralesional corticosteroid injections, following the protocol outlined by Terry and Jacoway. The injections were given on a weekly basis for six weeks. A mixture of 7 cm^3 of triamcinolone acetonide and 0.5 percent marcaine with 1/200,000 epinephrine (mixed in a 1:1 ratio) was injected intralesionally on the first and second appointments. On the third appointment, 6 cm^3 of the mixture was injected into the lesion. An increase in back pressure was noted on injection. At the fourth through sixth appointments, 6cm^3 of the corticosteroid mixture was injected into the lesion. During the last three treatments, they found that it was increasingly difficult to perforate the cortical bone for injections. An increase in the amount of back pressure in the syringe was noted during these treatments as well.

Panoramic radiographs obtained immediately after the sixth treatment showed early bone fill of the lesion. Subsequent radiographic evaluations at three and seven months after treatment continued to show good bone consolidation. A decrease in the buccal expansion was first noted at three months. By seven months, the patient's facial appearance had returned to normal, and they noted almost complete filling of the osteolytic area with new bone. Intraorally, some buccal expansion was still present.

They concluded that intralesinal corticosteroid injections was a good alternative to surgery in the treatment of CGCGs. The technique is simple and inexpensive and allows clinicians to spare vital structures, thus avoiding large defects of the jaws. They were surprised that this simple method of treating a potentially aggressive lesion has not found wide application.

Statistical evaluation of a large number of patients in a long-term prospective study is required to provide documentation and verification of the efficacy of this attractive nonsurgical modality.

TEMPOROMANDIBULAR JOINT PAIN AND DYSFUNCTION

Kopps et al (1985) conducted a comparative study to assess the short-term effect of intra-articular injections of Sodium Hyaluronate and a corticosteroid (betamethasone) in a sample of 33 patients who had pain and tenderness to palpation in the temporomanibular joint of at least six months duration that had not responded to previous conservative treatment. The two drugs were randomly allocated to superior joint compartment of the TMJ with a two-week interval between injections. The effect on subjective symptoms, clinical signs, and bite force was assessed. Both drugs reduced the symptoms and signs significantly, and no statistically significant difference between the drugs. They revealed that the difference between the drugs in terms of short-term therapeutic effects was small, and that sodium hyaluronate could be used as an alternative to corticosteroid for patients who have signs of TMJ inflammation, especially for those who have symptomatic osteoarthrosis.

Kopp S et al (1987) conducted a comparative study and the long-term effect of intra-articular injections of Sodium Hyaluronate and corticosteroid (betamethasone) in a sample of 24 patients who had pain and tenderness on palpation of the temporomandibular joint (TMJ arthritis) of at least six months duration, and who had not responded to conservative treatment. The two drugs were randomly allocated to the patients. The drugs 0.5ml, were injected twice into the superior joint compartment of the TMJ with a two-week interval between injections.

Sodium hyaluronate (10mg/ml) was dissolved in a phosphate buffer (pH 7.75) with added sodium chloride (Hylartil, Pharmacia AB, Uppsala). Equal amounts of the disodium-phosphate and acetate esters of betamethasone were used in a suspension of 6mg/ml (celestone bifas, Schering-Plough Corp., Kenilworth, NJ). The disodium phosphate ester of the drug was readily soluble and had an immediate effect, unlike the acetate ester that was difficult to dissolve and thereby had a prolonged effect.

The drugs were dispensed in sterile, disposable syringes and were injected with a 0.6mm diameter needle. The skin in the area was carefully washed with benzalkonium chloride (0.1%), iodine (5%), and alcohol (70%). A volume of 0.5ml of either drug was injected into the superior compartment of the TMJ with the mouth opened maximally.

At the one and two-year follow-ups both the hyaluronate and the corticosteroid-group had significantly reduced subjective symptoms as well as clinical signs, and the maximum voluntary bite force was significantly increased. The differences in effect between treatments were not statistically significant. It was concluded that both drugs have a significant long-term effect on chronic arthritis of the TMJ; however, sodium hyaluronate might be the best alternative due to the least risk of side effects.

Wenneberg B et al (1991) studied the long term development (2 and 8 years after treatment) of subjective and clinical dysfunction in the stomatognathic system as well as the radiographic appearance of the TMJ after three intraarticular corticosteroid injections.

16 patients with pain localized to the TMJ for at least 3 months and joint tenderness on palpation were chosen for the study. Patients whose symptoms could be referred to disease in other components of the stomatognathic system (eg, toothache, myalgia, neuralgia) were excluded. Second criterion was failure of previous conservative treatments (eg, occlusal adjustment occlusal splints, and / or physical exercises).

A mixture of 0.5ml of betamethasone (equal amounts of its disodium-phosphate and acetate esters) were used in a suspension of 6 mg/ml (Celestone bifas) and an equal volume of lidocaine-chloride-anhydrate (xylocaine, 10mg/ml) was injected into the superior joint compartment of the TMJ three times with an interval of 1 week between treatment. The effects were assessed before (visit I), 2 years after (visit II), and 8 years after treatment (visit III). All patients were examined and treated by one of two examiners, the same one on each occasion.

A multiple-choice questionnaire was used to assess the subjective symptoms.

Routine examination methods, including examination for tenderness on palpation of the TMJ (posteriorly and laterally) and masticatory muscle regions, TMJ sounds (clicking or crepitus), soft-tissue swelling over the TMJ, maximum movement capacity of the mandible, pain during mandibular movements, and deviation of the mandible during opening, were used.

Radiographic examination of the TMJ was performed before and 8 years after corticosteroid treatment.

The subjective symptoms as well as the clinical signs were significantly reduced at the follow-up examination. Erosions of the bony articular margins of the TMJ that could be observed radiographically before treatment were found to be remineralized at the follow-up and associated with bony remodeling (deviation in shape) of the joint. They reported that the long-term prognosis of intra-articular glucocorticosteroid injections for TMJ arthritis is good and that there are no radiographically demonstrable side effects of the treatment.

CHRONIC ULCERATIVE STOMATITIS :

Recently, a distinct new disease entity, chronic ulcerative stomatits (CUS), has been described in a limited number of case reports. CUS resembles erosive lichen planus or oral discoid lupus erythematosus in its clinical and histologic manifestations. Therefore, it is best diagnosed via immunofluorescence in conjunction with routine histopathology. DIF may reveal nuclear deposits of immunoglobulin G (IgG) in a speckled pattern mainly in the basal third of the epithelium. This may be coupled with deposits of fibrinogen in the basement membrane zone. This unique pattern of antinuclear antibody (ANA) has been referred to as stratified epithelium specific antinuclear antibody (SES-ANA).

Lorenzana ER, Rees TD, Glass M, Detweiler JG (2000)[52] reported a case of a 54 year-old woman who presented with a 2 to 3-year history of stomatitis and dry mouth. She stated that by eating anything spicy and fruit exacerbated her condition. She believed her condition to be associated with stress since she had just changed jobs and her daughter had just married. Her blood studies revealed slightly elevated cholesterol levels but otherwise, no significant findings.

Clinical examination revealed diffuse erythema along the right and left buccal mucosa, the facial attached gingiva in both arches, and over the incisive papilla of the palate. Plaque-like white lesions were also present bilaterally on the facial gingiva of the mandibular molars. A clinical diagnosis of erosive (atrophic) lichen planus was made. The histopathologic diagnosis of the buccal mucosa, was chronic mucositis with lichenoid features. The minor salivary gland biopsy revealed chronic sialadenitis with a Sjogren's syndrome grading scale IV.

The patient was given a prescription for fluocinonide, a 0.05% topical corticosteroid gel for use 4 times daily on the affected sites.

Following 3 weeks of treatment with fluocinonide, the patient reported that the lesions were less painful. Her medication was changed to betamethasone dipropionate, a 0.05% topical corticosteroid gel, 4 times daily, in an attempt to achieve remission. Two months after beginning the use of betamethasone dipropionate, the patient reported significant relief of the pain and using it again 2 weeks later, just prior to her scheduled recall. At the recall appointment, her gingiva showed little improvement, with erythema present in localized areas. Subsequently, however, complete remission of lesions was achieved and the patient was then able to discontinue betamethasone dipropionate therapy with instructions to reinitiate therapy, in the event lesions began to recur.

PYOSTOMATITIS VEGETANS :

Pyostomatitis vegetans, the occurrence of oral vegetations, pustules, and ulcers, is the oral equivalent of pyoderma vegetans. Oral and cutaneous lesions are similar and may be seen concurrently or in isolation. The association of pyostomatitis vegetans with gastrointestinal disease is well established. Ulcerative colitis is the most common association, but other forms of colitis may be associated. The oral manifestations of ulcerative colitis may include not only pyostomatitis vegetans but also aphthoid hemorrhagic ulcers.

Chan SWY et al (1991) reported a case of a 23-year old white man who had a 6-month history of oral ulceration. No malaise or pyrexia were present. His medical history revealed that ulcerative colitis had been diagnosed when he was 21 years old. This diagnosis had been confirmed by sigmoidoscopy and rectal biopsy, and he was being treated with corticosteroid enemas and intermittent therapy with sulfasalazine.

On examination no cutaneous, genital, or ocular lesions were present. Lymphadenopathy was absent, but the patient appeared wasted and tired. Oral examination revealed ulcers on the buccal mucosa, lower labial mucosa, palate, uvula, and floor of the mouth. The labial ulcer closely resembled a snail-track ulcer.

Hematologic investigations revealed a lowered serum ferritin level and elevated IgM level and serum electrophoresis showed an increase in the acute-phase protein α_2–globulin. An oral biopsy showed epithelial acantholysis and intraepithelial abscess formation consistent with pyostomatitis vegetans. Direct immunofluorescence was positive for IgG and C3 in the basement membrane zone, but indirect immune fluorescence was negative.

The patient was subsequently prescribed ferrous sulfate and betamethasone mouthrinse for 2 months. The oral lesions were monitored regularly. At one stage an exacerbation of the oral lesions warranted the systemic use of prednisolone (20 mg for 2 days, 15mg for 1 day, 10 mg for 1 day, and 5mg for 1 day); this was further supplemented with a tetracycline mouthwash.

A year later the patient had another exacerbation with ulcers and vegetations affecting the labial gingivae and the lower labial mucosa, and increased gastrointestinal symptoms. The gingival lesions consisted of rosettes of small ulcers and vegetation. Sulfasalazine was again used to control the gastrointestinal condition ; this was followed by the resolution of the oral lesions within a few months.

HEMANGIOMA :

Hemangiomas are vascular malformations which occur at birth. They are more common in females in a ratio of 2:1. More than half the cases are noted clinically before the first decade of life. They appear on skin as macular areas red to pink to blue and somtimes as elevated lesions with bruit. They appear to grow up to puberty and then stop growing. Kasabach-Merritt syndrome is characterized by the association of a rapidly enlarging hemangioma with thrombocytopenia, purpura, haemorrhagic diathesis, microangiopathic hemolytic anemia and consumptive coagulopathy.

Takato T, Komuro Y, Yonehara Y (1993) reported a case of an infant with a giant parotid hemangioma associated with KMS (Kasabach Merritt syndrome). The tumor had been present at birth and had subsequently rapidly enlarged. Examination revealed a large (5 x 6-cm), firm, purplish red mass that was neither fluctuant nor pulsatile. Laboratory data indicating a severe consumption coagulopathy. A computed tomography (CT) scan showed a large swelling of the left parotid gland.

At 44 days of age, daily prednisone therapy (8mg/d) was begun. Simultaneously, the left parotid region was irradiated daily with 9 MeV, to a total dose of 15 Gy (11 fractions). Irradiation ended at 60 days of age. A progressive increase in hemoglobin and platelet count to normal and regression of the tumor occurred during the 19 days following the treatment. Follow-up at 8 years showed resolution of the residual hemangioma, without facial nerve dysfunction nor facial bone asymmetry. A CT scan showed symmetrical parotid glands. Radiotherapy (15 Gy) combined with prednisone (2mg/kg/d) was used to treat this infant and undoubtedly contributed to the improvement in terms of tumor shrinkage and thrombocytopenia that occurred. No complications as a result of the radiotherapy was observed to date.

MIESCHER'S GRANULOMATOUS CHEILITIS :

Granulomatous cheilitis (GC), a rare disorder of unknown etiology, is characterized by nonremissive enlargement of one or both lips with typical granulomatous findings on histologic examination. GC is considered by some authors to be a monosymptomatic form of Melkersson-Rosenthal syndrome (MRS) and has also been associated with sarcoidosis, Crohn's disease, gingival granulomatosis, and Anderson-Fabry disease.

Hernandez G, Hernandez F and Lucas M (1986) reported a case of a 26-year-old white woman presented because of a massive, unsightly enlargement of the upper lip. About 18 months prior to the visit, she had noticed the sudden onset of progressively increasing indolent edema of the upper lip. The swelling was not related to any particular cause and, at times, produced a feeling of tightness. She reported that occasionally the edema partially receded during the evening. She was initially treated by a dermatologist, who found positive reactions to lactalbumin, nuts, and rye on allergy testing. A hypoallergenic diet was prescribed, and the patient was given gamma globulin injections and oral triamcinolone. This therapeutic trial was unsuccessful. Results of physical examination were essentially normal, except for exaggerated enlargement of the upper lip. The oral mucosa, teeth, gums, tongue, and salivary glands were normal. Results of neurologic examination were also normal. The laboratory tests performed included complete blood count; erythrocyte sedimentation rate: calcium, phosphate, electrolyte, total protein, uric acid, and creatinine levels; liver function tests; and serum determinations of immunoglobulins C'3c, C'4, and sterase C'1 inhibitor. All results were within normal limits. The radiographic study of the maxillofacial area did not show any abnormality. The allergy tests showed hypersensitivity to almonds and hazelnuts (lactalbumin and other dry fruits had been positive previously). The clinical diagnosis was granulomatous cheilitis. A biopsy was performed under local anesthesia. The histologic diagnosis was granulomatous cheilitis.

Treatment consisted of submucosal injections of 0.5ml (3mg/ml) of betamethasone (betamethasone acetate-betamethasone disodium phosphate), once a week for two consecutive weeks, followed by two injections every four months, during a 16-month period. The enlargement of the lip had almost disappeared after 30 days of this treatment. The patient had a recurrence of the edema coincident with the ingestion of almonds and tunafish five months later, once again requiring two injections of betamethasone. After this second episode, the enlargement decreased, except for the philtrum area. The treatment was discontinued, and the patient was symptom-free after 10 months.

USES IN ORAL SURGERY:

Laskin DM, Giglio JA (2001) reviewed the therapeutic uses of corticosteroids in oral and maxillofacial surgery. Various treatments are available to improve patient comfort and relieve the anxiety associated with oral and maxillofacial surgical procedures. These interventions work at selected points along the path from surgical injury to the patient's perception and reaction to the painful stimuli and are summarized as :

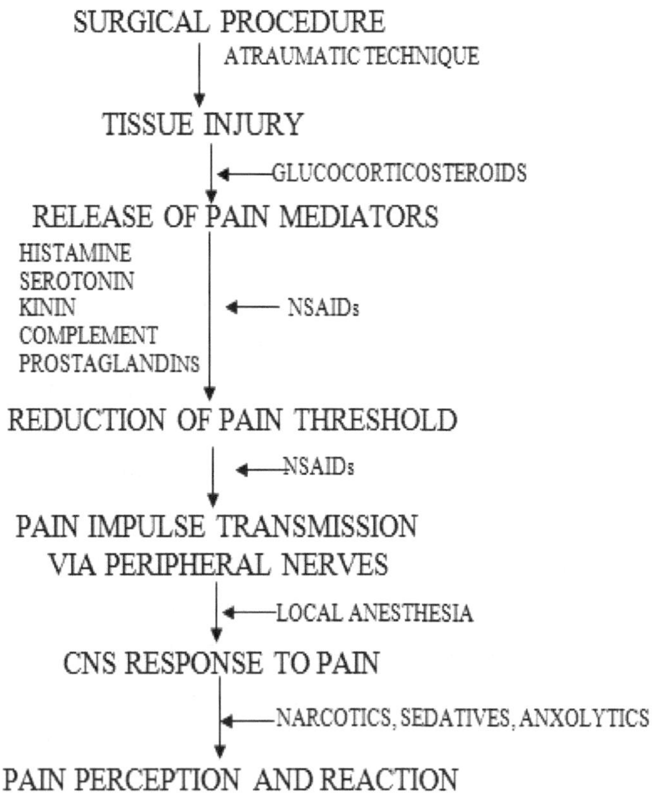

The inhibitory effects of glucocorticosteroids on inflammation and edema constitute the basis for this therapeutic efficacy and their principal use in oral and maxillofacial surgery. Steroids have been used after varied procedures such as third molar removal; reconstructive surgery; preprosthetic surgery, including lowering the floor of the mouth; and vestibuloplasty with a palatal graft. No standard regimens or protocols for drug dosing or route of administration have been developed, however.

Third molar surgery :

In a placebo-controlled study, Beirne and Hollander administered 125 mg of methylprednisolone intravenously before third molar surgery and compared postoperative pain, swelling, and trismus between placebo and active drug groups. Significantly less pain and swelling were reported with methylprednisolone than with placebo, but no statistically significant difference in trismus was noted between groups.

Hooley JR, Hohl TH (1974) Hooley and Francis (1969) advocated the oral use of betamethasone for the reduction of swelling, trismus, and indirectly pain after the difficult removal of mandibular third molars. In their study, they found that patients in the control group had significantly more edema and twice as much trismus and required twice as much medication for pain as the group that received betamethasone.

Francis' regimen originally was two 0.6mg tablets the evening before surgery, and two 0.6mg tablets four times a day on the day of surgery and thereafter until expiration of the prescription. The total dosage did not exceed 24 tablets or 14.4 mg. To eliminate the need for oral medication postoperatively, Francis has modified his regimen to incorporate the use of the intramuscular form of betamethasone. This intramuscular suspension consisted of equal parts of betamethasone sodium phosphate and betamethasone acetate. The current regimen consists of two 0.6mg tablets the evening before surgery, one 0.6mg tablet the morning of surgery, and 6 mg of betamethasone intramuscularly at the time of surgery.

Senders CW et al (1999) studied the effects of periopertive steroid therapy on pediatric patients who underwent primary palatoplasty. They found that perioperative steroid therapy (IV dexamethasone sodium phosphate, 0.25 mg / kg, immediately preoperatively and once every 8 hours for two doses postoperatively) significantly reduced the incidence of postoperative airway distress and fever. Postoperative fluid intake, discharge eligibility, and palatal fistula formation were not affected significantly. They concluded that these findings favour a customary role for perioperative steroid therapy in pediatric primary palatoplasty.

One of the indications has been is in the management of temporomandibular joint (TMJ) disorders, where it has been used by intraarticular injection, IM injection, iontophoresis, and phonophoresis. In patients with an acute episode of osteoarthritis of the TMJ who have not responded to NSAID therapy, the intraarticular injection of a glucocorticosteroid has been shown to provide relief of the subjective symptoms and the clinical signs in the joint, which may be long-lasting in some patients. It also has been found have to have a short-term effect in patients with rheumatoid arthritis in the TMJ. Although a single injection may have a beneficial effect in selected patients, with osteoarthritis or rheumatoid arthritis, however, it has been shown that multiple injections may be harmful to the joint structures, and no more than three injections at a minimal interval of 1 to 3 months are recommended.

The IM injunction of a steroid, alone or in combination with local anesthesia, also has been used to treat the trigger points and muscles spasm associated with myofascial pain and dysfunction in the muscles or mastication. It has been shown that local anesthetic agents other than procaine can produce long-term muscle damage and that this is increased by the addition of a steroid.

Reconstructive oral surgery : Edema, following the procedures such as the sagittal osteotomy of the mandible can be of such extreme proportion that tracheostomy is required to maintain the patency of the airway. While swelling of that magnitude is rare, extreme swelling after sagittal osteotomy must be considered common.

Messer UJ, and Keller JJ (1975) advocated the use of intraoral dexamethasone after the extraction of mandibular third molars. Upon completion of surgical procedures, 4 mg of dexamethasone was administered intramuscularly into the masseter muscle using a specified technique. Dexamethasone has equipotent anti-inflammatory activity to betamethasone and lacks much of the sodium-retaining properties of hydrocortisone. These investigators considered that the use of dexamethasone, as described, produced a predictable decrease in a total lack of, post-operative pain, the decrease in oedema and trismus was based on clinical observations in the immediate post-operative days.

Caci F and Gluck GM (1976) reported on a double blind study of prednisolone and papase as inhibitors of complications after oral surgery. Prednisolone is a synthetic analogue of cortisol, with a dose of 20 mg possessing an equivalent anti-inflammatory potency to 80 mg of cortisol. Papase is a proteolytic enzyme and it has been suggested that it is effective in eliminating the cellular components of inflammation. Prednisolone 5 mg and papase were used on 129 patients. The post-surgical course was evaluated relative to oedema, trismus and pain. A comparison of patients treated with prednisolone, papase and a placebo indicated no significant difference for oedema; however, significant differences were found for trismus and pain ($P<0.05$). The authors considered that the lack of difference found with regard to oedema could be attributable to the fact that relatively few observed within 4 days post-operatively. Prednisolone was found to be more effective in reducing trismus and pain than papase.

Huffman GG (1977) suggested the use of methylprednisolone sodium succinate to reduce post-operative oedema after removal of impacted third molars. The equivalent anti-inflammatory dose of methylprednisolone as compared with 80 mg of hydrocortisone is 16 mg. In this investigation, 129 patients were placed into 3 groups. Group 1 (44 patients) acted as the control; group 2 (42 patients) were given 40 mg of methylprednisolone intravenously immediately preoperatively and group 3 (43 pateints) received 125 mg of methylprednisolone intra-venously immediately pre-operatively. The patients were examined on the 1st, 2nd and 7th post-operative days. The degree of swelling was rated by visual inspection and palpation. There was a statistically significant reduction in the post-operative oedema in those patients given methylprednisolone ($P<0.005$) at both 24 and 48 h post-operatively. There was no statistical significance in the findings between the 40 mg and 120 mg doses. At the end of a week, there was an insignificant difference between all 3 groups.

Seymour RA, Walton JG (1984) reported the effect of betamethasone after bilateral lower third molar removal. Betamethasone has a more potent anti-inflammatory action than hydrocortisone, the equivalent anti-inflammatory doses being 3 mg and 80 mg respectively. Patients received 2 betamethasone tablets (0.6 mg in each tablet), or an identical placebo, on the evening prior to surgery, followed by the same dose 4 times a day on the day of surgery and for the subsequent 2 days. A photographic method was used to measure and quantitatively assess the degree of post-operative swelling. Pain was assessed by comparing the patient's analgesic consumption after treatment with betamethasone and placebo. Tetracycline cones were inserted into all extraction sockets.

Information was collected from 47 patients and it was found that betamethasone profoundly affected the post-operative oedema, the control group had about 6 tiems as much oedema as the betamethasone group. There was also a significant reduction in the amount of trismus, to less than half. The incidence of alveolar osteitis (dry socket) was higher in the betamethasone group than in the control group, but even then it was only 4%. These investigators considered that the administration of steroid preparations, such as betamethasone, for a short period is a safe procedure.

Sisk AL, Bonnington GJ (1985) evaluated the efficacies of corticosteroids therapy and nonsteroidal anti-inflammatory agent therapy for the reduction of the acute postoperative inflammatory response and its undesirable sequelae of pain edema, and trismus. Comparison was made of parenteral corticosteroids therapy, oral nonsteroidal anti-inflammatory agent therapy, and oral non-antiinflammatory analgesic therapy.

Sixty patients, each in need of extraction of four impacted third molars, who met strict clinical and radiographic criteria concerning tooth position and anticipated degree of difficulty of extractions were selected. No clinical or radiographic evidence of infection or inflammation was permitted around any of the proposed surgical sites.

No anti-inflammatory medications, including aspirin, were permitted for at least 10 days prior to the surgical procedures.

Each subject received, on a random basis one of the three agents under evaluation.

Baseline pain-assessment scales consisted of a four-point category rating scale (no pain, mild pain, moderate pain, severe pain) and a 100-mm horizontal visual analog scale, with the left end of the scale labeled "no pain" and the right end labeled "pain as much as it could be".

Thirty minutes before the start of surgery each patient received either flurbiprofen, 2 mg, or an identical-appearing placebo tablet, both administrated orally with a small sip of water.

Immediately following administration of the local anesthetic, a single 125-mg dose of the corticosteroid methylprednisolone or an equal amount in volume of an identical appearing placebo was administrated, intravenously over a 1-minute period. The four third molar teeth were then removed by a standard surgical technique.

Patients in the nonsteroidal anti-inflammatory group were supplied with 16-50-mg tablets of flurbiprofen and were instructed to ingest one of these tablets every 6 hours until all 16 had been taken.

The results of this study appeared to indicate that a single class of drugs is not maximally effective in controlling both postoperative pain and postoperative swelling. Flubriprofen (a nonsteroidal anti-inflammatory agent) is an effective analgesic, while methylprednisolone (a corticosteroid) had little analgesic activity. Methylprednisolone is more effective than flurbiprofen in control of postsurgical swelling, while neither drug appeared to be effective in controlling. Postoperative trismus. A combination of these two medications may be necessary to control the sequelae of oral surgical procedures most effectively.

Mosgaw SS, Schmelzeisen R, Frolich JC et al (1995) conduced a study to test a combination treatment of ibuprofen and methylprednisolone for pain and swelling.

The efficacy of 32 mg methylprednisolone on pain and swelling when given 12 hours before and after surgery in combination with 400 mg ibuprofen three times a day given immediately on the day of the operation and investigated in a placebo-controlled, intraindividual double-blind study.

After use of ibuprofen/methylprednisolone, ultrasonic examination showed a reduction in swelling of 56% (P<.001) compared with the placebo group; measurement with a tape measure showed a 58% (P<.001) reduction in swelling. The visual analog scale showed a reduction of 67.7% in postoperative pain in comparison with placebo.

They concluded that the combination of ibuprofen and methylprednisolone had good analgesic and anti-inflammatory action.

Flood TR, McMAnners J, Atter A et al (1999) conducted study to find out if giving steroids reduced postoperative swelling in orbital surgery. 20 patients who required orbital floor exploration after injuires were selected. Patients were given methylprednisolone 250 mg (or placebo identically packaged) at induction of anaesthesia, with a further three doses at 6-hourly intervals postoperatively. Differences in interpalpebral width before and after operation were noted. Those given steroids (n=11) had a signifanctly increased interpalpebral width compared with placebo (n=9) postoperatively (P<0.01, 95%

confidence intervals of the difference = 1 mm-6mm). They concluded that short courses of steroid therapy should be considered in orbital surgery for appropriate patients. There was an advantage in being able to assess the globe postoperatively.

Esen E, Tasar F, Akhan O (1999) evaluated the anti-inflammatory effect and adrenal suppressive side effect of methylprednisolone sodium succinate (MP) on the postoperative sequelae of third molar surgery using objective methods in a double-blind, crossover study.

Twenty patients who were to undergo surgical removal of bilateral, symmetrically placed lower third molars were studied. Each patient was given 125 mg MP intravenously before surgery on one side, and a placebo before surgery on the opposite side on a random basis. Ultrasonographic and computed tomographic examinations were performed to determine the amount of facial edema. Trismus was evaluated by measuring maximal interincisal opening, and pain was evaluated by recording the number of standard analgesic tablets used on the day of surgery and the first postoperative day. Hypothalamic-pituitary-adrenal (HPA) axis function was tested by measuring basal plasma cortisol stimulation test also was performed before and after administration of MP, to evaluate adrenal function.

Statistical analysis of the data indicated a significant decrease in edema, trismus, and pain in the MP group. Plasma cortisol levels showed a nonsignificant decrease in both the MP- and placebo-treated groups. The ACTH stimulation test indicated normal HPA axis function before and after MP administration. No clinically apparent infection, disturbance of wound healing, or other corticosteroid-related complications were noted. Eighteen patients (90%) indicated a preference for the overall postoperative course when MP was used.

In the absence of contraindications for corticosteroid administration, preoperative use of MP appeared to be a safe and effective method of reducing postoperative complications in third molar surgery.

Preprosthetic surgery :

Hall DH (1971) has suggested the use of dexamethasone in conjuction with the buccal vestibuloplasty with palatal graft and lowering of the floor of the mouth. His regimen was similar to that suggested by Guernsey and DeChamplain. He noticed excellent results after the use of dexamethasone in major preprosthetic surgery. In addition to decreasing edema, it has also made possible the early discharge of patients from the hospital.

Guernsey LH and DeChamplain RW (1971) Their regimen consisted of dexamethasone, 4 mg on the night before surgery, 4 mg twice a day on the day of surgery, 2 mg twice a day on the first postoperative day and 1 mg on the second and third postoperative days. This regimen significantly reduced postoperative edema and that it has contributed to a distinct decrease in the average hospital stay of these patients.

Adjunctive use : Topical steroids aid in the prevention of ulcerations and excoriations of the lips and corners of the mouth after retraction of these tissues. It is a practice to liberally apply a topical steroid such as fluocinolone acetonide, 0.025%, or a mixture of hydrocortisone, 1%, and dexpanthenol, 2%, to the lips and corners of the mouth during major surgical orthodontic and preprosthetic procedures.

ENDODONTICS

Krasner P, Jackson E (1986) reported the use of orally administered dexamethasone alone for the management of pain following routine endodontic instrumentation.

Before beginning treatment, patients were asked to rate their pain on a 0 to 100 scale, where 0 means "no pain" and 100 means "greatest possible pain".

All subjects received the following first-appointment endodontic treatment : the pulp chamber was completely unroofed, a canal length measurement was determined by radiograph, all canals were filed with 10, 15, and 20 K-type files while copiously irrigating with 2.5% sodium hypochlorite, and the access was sealed with a sterile cotton pellet (no medicament) and Cavit. All subjects were treated by the same endodontist. At the end of the appointment, each subject was given seven tablets in a coded envelope and instructed to take three immediately and then one tablet every 3 hours until bedtime. Twenty-five subjects, randomly selected, received tablets that contained 0.75 mg of dexamethasone; the remaining twenty-five subjects received placebos.

Statistical analysis was done and the results showed that the subjects receiving dexamethasone reporting less pain than the subjects receiving placebos.

Few side effects were reported like dizziness, stomach upset, swelling of the face, and tachycardia. None of these effects was considered to be severe enough to discontinue the prescribed medication.

In the present study, posttreatment endodontic pain was substantially reduced by administration of oral dexamethasone.

Chance K, Lin L, Shovlin FE (1987) conducted a study to evaluate in a double-blind manner the ability of intracanal corticosteroid to relieve postoperative pain during endodontic therapy.

Three-hundred endodontic patients in the department were randomly entered into the study. Patients were excluded from the study if active suppurative lesions were present.

Test and control solutions were prepared and transferred into identical sterile vials containing a numerical identification. The vials were prepared by a second investigator not involved in the clinical aspect of the study. The test solution contained prednisolone acetate (2.5%) in an aqueous suspension obtained as a commercial preparation. The control solution contained sterile normal saline.

A standard technique was used for the coronal access preparation. Length determination to the radiographic apex was obtained, and the radicular cavity preparation was accomplished by using the step-back technique. The minimum diameter of the apical one-third of each prepared canal was equivalent to a standard #25 K file. Test or control solutions were placed into the canal to the working length (radiographic apex) by means of sterile paper points saturated with either solution. Each application was repeated three times with the paper point remaining in place for at least 10 s. The paper point was then removed and the pulp canal left patent. A sterile cotton pellet moistened with aqueous parachlorophenol (2%) and squeezed dry was used to cover the canal orifices and the access cavity was sealed to a 3 to 4 mm depth with cavit.

After 24 h the patient was seen in person or contacted by telephone. Those who experienced pain were contacted every 24 h until the symptoms subsided. The experience of the patient was recorded in one of four categories ; no pain, slight pain but no medication required, moderate pain that required a mild analgesic and severe pain that required a narcotic.

Only four patients (2.7%) in the experimental group required posttreatment narcotic medication, an opening of the involved tooth for drainage, or both. Nine patients (6.8%) in the control group required the same type of treatment. When compared with the control group, the reduced incidence of severe pain in the experimental group was significant) $p = 0.05$).

Regardless of treatment, pain dissipated within 24 h in 69 of 123 (56.1%) patients. The difference between treatment groups of pain lasting less or more than 24 h was not significant.

Pain occurred more frequently in the control group than in the experimental group when vital pulps were extirpated. This finding was statistically significant at p=0.007. However, when the pulp was nonvital before treatment, the difference was not significant.

The corticosteroid was effective in significantly reducing the incidence of postoperative pain in teeth where vital pulp was present. However, when the pulp was necrotic, the corticosteroid was ineffective in reducing the incidence of postoperative pain.

Erisen R, Yucel T, Kucukay S et al (1989) reported a case of hypoesthesia caused by endomethasone overflowing into the mandibular canal. 13 year old boy, who stated that he had undergone root canal treatment in his left lower first molar. He reported with pain and complainted of swelling. During the clinical examination, a swelling around the first molar, which extended between the vestibule and angulus mandibulae, was observed. On control radiographs, an overflow of the filling material was encountered. Contact with the dentist who performed the endodontic treatment, revealed that endomethasone was employed as the root canal filling material.

Fachin EVF, Zaki AE (1991) conducted a study to histologically investigate steroid effects on the dental pulp. Three steroid preparations, hydrocortisone, betamethasone and triamcinolone, were locally applied to the exposed pulp tissue in rat incisors after pulpectomy. After 24 hrs the effects on the tissues were assessed by light microscopy. The results showed that topical application of corticosteroids as an intracanal medicament reduced inflammatory changes in the pulp as compared with controls. furthermore, triamcinolone and betamethasone demonstrated more potent anti-inflammatory effects than did hydrocortisone.

Tjaderhane LS, Pajari UH, Ahola RH et al (1995) studied the effects of different kinds of emergency treatments on flare-ups and other related complications. A total of 197 teeth received emergency treatment after diagnosis at the beginning of the root canal therapy; in 103 the pulp chamber was left open for drainage of pus, 35 were treated with dexamethasone sodium phosphate, and 59 with various other medicaments, followed by routine root canal treatment, including chloramphenicol (Klorita, Laake-Farmos Inc, Turkyu, Finland), 1% chlorhexidine or calcium hydroxide. Chloramphenicol, dexamethasone and chlorhexidine were applied to the root canal with pipettes, calcium hydroxide with a lentulo spiral filler. Another 404 teeth received root canal treatment without prior emergency treatment. If symptoms occurred during treatment, flare-up was said to be present. If a periapical radiolucency was found, long-term calcium hydroxide treatment was used. No sign of periapical healing radiographically after 6 months was described as a complication. The percentage of teeth with no complications varied from 72.2% (dexamethasone) to 78.9% (other modification) and the results showed no differences between the groups in the teeth with no complications, flare-ups or other complications. The number of bacteria detected with Gram's staining was higher in the teeth which were left open. In conclusion, leaving the pulp chamber open for drainage had no effect on the incidence of flare-ups or other complications.

Gerosa R, Menegazzi G, Borin M et al (1995) evaluated the toxicity of six different endodontic cements: AH-26, Pulp Canal Sealer, Rocanal-R2, rocanal-R3, Bioseal, and Endomethasone. The toxicity was determined by measuring spectrophotometrically at 405 nm the colorimetric reaction of N-acetyl-β-hexosaminidase, and endogenous enzyme, with the chromogenic substrate (p-nitrophenol-N-acetyl-β-D-glucosamide (NAG)). Severe cytotoxicity was observed in the 1 and 2 week test solutions of AH-26. pulp canal sealer and endomethasone showed low cytotoxicity in the 1 and 2 week test solutions at 24, 48 and 72 h. Moderate cytotoxicity was observed in the 1 and 2 week test solutions of bioseal, except at 48 and 72 h, and in the 2 week test solutions at 24, 48 and 72 h. moderate cytotoxicity was seen in the 1 and 2 week test solutions of rocanal-R3 only at 24 h. The aim of this study was to evaluate the toxicity of six different endodontic sealers, most frequently used in our clinical practice. Endomethasone contains hydrocortisone, which can contribute to its toxicity.

*

CONCLUSION

In conclusion, corticosteroids are medicines that are similar to the natural hormone cortisol and belong to the family of drugs called steroids. These drugs have wide spread effects, which include action on body's metabolism, inflammatory processes and immune system. They are often used in treating skin problem, severe allergies, asthma and arthritis. These drugs are also used among patients who have recieved organ transplants, to reduce the chance or rejection and other immune mediated pathologies.

Corticosteroids now a days come in a variety of sources, suitable for treating different conditions. Though these drugs are useful in treating many medical conditions they also have many undesirable side effects. These side effects are rare when used for a short time. The major side effect is, they may lower the body's ability to fight off infections or may make infections harder to treat. Other common side effecs include changes in appetite (increase or decrease), nervousness, restlessness, sleep problem, indigestion and osteoporosis.

Thus we as oral diagnosticians should weigh the advantages and disadvantages prior to prescription of corticosteroids.

*

REFERENCES

1) Acton CHC. Steroid-induced anterior open bite. Case report. Aus Dent Journal 1986; 31 (6): 455-8.
2) Addy M, Pimlott SJ, Thaw M. The oral retention of prednisolone mouthwashes – effects of concenteration and time. J Oral Med 1986; 41(2): 82-86.
3) Adornato MC, Paticoff KA. Intralesional corticosteroid injection for treatment of central giant-cell granuloma. JADA 2001; 132: 186-190.
4) Allen CM, Camisa C. Paraneoplastic pemphigus: a review of the literature. Oral diseases. 2000;6: 208-214.
5) Bahn SL. Corticosteroids in Dentistry. JADA 1982; 105 : 476 – 481.
6) Bailoor DN, Nagesh KS, Reddi R. Oral Precancer. In: Fundamentals of Oral Medicine and Radiology. Authors: Bailoor DN, Nagesh KS. Codeword Process And Printers, Mangalore.2nd ed. 2001: 281- 296.
7) Bailoor DN, Nagesh KS. Salivary Gland Disorders. In: Fundamentals of Oral Medicine and Radiology. Codeword Process And Printers, Mangalore.2nd ed. 2001: 315- 340.
8) Boyd AS, Neldner KH. Lichen planus. J Am Acad Dermatol 1991; 25: 593-619.

9) Brice DM, Danesh-Meyer MJ. Oral lesions in patients with psoriasis : clinical presentation and management. J Periodontol 2000; 71(12): 1896-1903.

10) Brook IM, Noort RV, Pandurangi AV et al (1991)23 Controlled intraoral delivery of hydrocortisone sodium succinate. Oral Surg Oral Med Oral Pathol 1991; 71: 435-9.

11) Buajeeb W, Kraivaphan P, Pobrurksa C et al. Efficacy of topical retinoic acid compared with topical fluocinolone acetonide in the treatment of oral lichen planus. Oral Surg Oral Med Oral Pathol Oral Radiol Endod 1997; 83: 21-5.

12) Carbone M, Conrotto D, Carrozzo M et al. topical corticosteroids in association with miconazole and chlorhexidine in the long-term management of atrophic-erosive oral lichen planus: a placebo-controlled and comparative study between clobetasol and fluocinonide. Oral Diseases 1999; 5: 44-49.

13) Carrozzo M, Gandolfo S. The management of oral lichen planus. Oral Diseases 1999; 5: 196-205.

14) Chainani-Wu N, Silverman Jr S, Lozanda F et al. Oral lichen planus patient profile, disease progression and treatment responses. JADA 2001; 132: 901-908.

15) Chan SWY et al. Pyostomatitis vegetans: Oral manifestation of ulcerative colitis. Oral Surg Oral Med Oral Pathol 1991; 72: 689-92.

16) Chance K, Lin L, Shovlin FE. Clinical trial of intracanal corticosteroid in root canal therapy. J Endodontics 1987; 13 (9): 466-468.

17) Chatra LK, Bailoor DN, John A. Clinical Pharmacology- Corticosteroids in Dentistry. In: Fundamentals of Oral Medicine and Radiology. Authors: Bailoor DN, Nagesh KS. Codeword Process And Printers, Mangalore.2nd ed. 2001: 605- 610.

18) Chaudhary SK. The Suprarenal Glands. In: Concise medical Physiology.New Central Book Agency (P) Ltd. Calcutta: 2nd ed.1995: 303- 315.

19) Chen H, Shih C, Yen KL et al. Facial candida albicans cellulites occurring in a patient with oral submucous fibrosis and unknown diabetes mellitus after local corticosteroid injection treatment. J Oral Pathol Med 2004; 33: 243-5.

20) Cohen DM, Bhattacharyya I. Cinnamon-induced oral erythema multiforme like sensitivity reaction. JADA, 2000; 131: 929.

21) Cooke BED. Recurrent mikulicz's aphthae treated with topical hydrocortisone hemisuccinate sodium-double-blind controlled clinical trial. Br Med Journal: 1960; 764-766.

22) Corticosteroids. 7th March 2002; Available at: http://www.ehendrick.org/healthy/00044060.html.

23) Crouch HR. The Endocrine System. In: Functional Human Anatomy. Churchill Livingstone; 2nd ed 1982: 584-587

24) Deb AC. Hormones. In: Fundamentals of biochemistry. New Central Book Agency (P) Ltd, Calcutta: 1st ed.1984: 400- 422.

25) Delange WE, Doorenbos H. Hormones and synthetic substitutes. In: Side effects of drugs. Authors: Meyler L and Herrheimer A.Churchill Livingstone.1970: 383-405.

26) Erisen R, Yucel T, Kucukay S et al: Endomethasone root canal filling material in the mandibular canal. Oral Surg Oral Med Oral Path 1989; 68 (3): 343-345.

27) Esen E, Tasar F, Akhan O. Determination of the anti-inflammatory effects of methylprednisolone on the sequelae of third molar surgery. Oral Maxillofac Surg. 1999; 57: 1201-1206.

28) Fachin EVF, Zaki AE: Histology and lysosomal cytochemistry of the postsurgically inflamed dental pulp after topical application of steroids. I. Histological study. Journal of Endodontics 1991; 17 (9): 457-60.

29) Flood TR, McManners J, Attar A et al. Randomized prospective study of the influence of steroids on postoperative eye opening after exploration of the orbital floor. Br J Oral and Maxillofac Surg. 1999; 37: 312-315.

30) Gerosa R, Menegazzi G, Borin M et al: Cytotoxicity evaluation of six root canal sealers. J Endo 1995; 21 (9): 446-448.

31) Gersema L, Pharm D, Baker K. Use of corticosteroids in oral surgery. J Oral Maxillofac surg 1992; 50 : 270-277.

32) Glick M. Glucorticosteroid replacement therapy: A literature review and suggested replacement therapy. Oral Surg Oral Med Oral Pathol 1989; 67: 614-20.

33) Gold SI. Root canal calcification associated with prednisone therapy: a case report. JADA 1989; 119: 523-525.

34) Gorsky M, Raviv M, Moskona D et al. clinical characteristics and treatment of patients with oral lichen planus in Israel. Oral Surg Oral Med Oral Pathol Oral Radiol Endod 1996; 82: 644-9.

35) Goth A. Adrenal steroids. In: Medical pharmacology. A Lange Medical Book 8th edition; 1972: 543-556.

36) Greenberg MS. Herpesvirus infections. Dent Clin North America 1996; 40(2): 359-369.

37) Gupta D, Sharma SC. Oral submucous fibrosis – a new treatment regimen. J Oral maxillofac surg 1988; 46: 830-833.

38) Guyton AC.Endocrinology and Reproduction. In: Textbook of medical physiology 8th ed 808- 936.

39) Hernandez G, Hernandez F, Lucas M. Miescher's granulomatous cheilitis: Literature review and report of a case. J Oral Maxillofac surg 1986; 44: 474-478.

40) Hooley JR, Hohl. Use of steroids in the prevention of some complications after traumatic oral surgery. J Oral Surg 1974; 32: 864-866.

41) Kalkarf KL, Hinrichs JE, Shaw DH. Management of the dental patients receiving corticoid medications. Oral surg 1982; 54(4): 396-400.

42) Keele CA, Neel E, Joels N. The Adrenal Glands. In: Samson Wright's Applied Physiology, Oxford University Press: 13th ed.1985: 529- 537.

43) Kermer C, Millesi W, Watzke IM. Local injection of corticosteroids for central giant cell granuloma. Int J Oral Maxillofac Surg 1994; 23: 366-368.

44) Konstantinidis AB, Markopoulos A, Trigonides G. Ampicillin induced erythema multiforme. J Oral Med 1985; 40 (4): 168.

45) Kopp S, Carlsson G, Haraldson T et al. Long-term effect of intra-articular injections of sodium Hyaluronate and corticosteroid on temporomandibular joint arthritis. J Oral Maxillofac surg 1987; 45: 929-935.

46) Kopps S, Wenneberg B, Haraldson T et al. The short-term effect of intra-articular injections of sodium Hyaluronate and corticosteroid on temporomandibular joint pain and dysfunction. J Oral Maxillofac surg 1985; 429-435.

47) Koteeswaran D, Bailoor DN, John A. Vesiculo-Bullous and Ulcerative Lesions of Oral Mucosa. In: Fundamentals of Oral Medicine and Radiology. Authors: Bailoor DN, Nagesh KS. Codeword Process And Printers, Mangalore.2nd ed. 2001: 205- 225.

48) Krasner P, Jackson E : Management of posttreatment endodontic pain with oral dexamethasone : A double-blind study. Oral Surg. Oral Med. Oral Pathol. 1986; 62: 187-190.

49) Lai DR, Chen HR, Lin LM et al. Clinical evaluation of different treatment methods for oral submucous fibrosis. A 10-year experience with 150 cases. J Oral Pathol Med 1995; 24: 402-6.

50) Laskin MD, Giglio AJ. The use of steroids and nonsteroidal anti-inflammatory drugs in oral and maxillofacial surgery. Oral and maxillofac surg clin of north America 2001; 13: 31- 41.

51) Laurence DR, Bennett PN. Endocrinology I: adrenal corticosteroids, antagonists, corticotrophin. In: Clinical Pharmacology, Churchill Livingstone: London 19th ed. 2002: 667- 677.

52) Lorenzana ER, Rees TD, Glass M, et al. Chronic ulcerative stomatitis: a case report. J Period 2000; 71(1): 104-111.

53) Lozada F, Silverman S, Cram D. Pemphigus vulgaris: A study of six cases treated with levamisole and prednisone. Oral surgery 1982; 54:(2) 161-165.

54) Lozada F, Silverman S, Migliorati C. Adverse side effects associated with prednisone in the treatment of patients with oral inflammatory ulcerative diseases. JADA 1984; 109: 269-270.

55) Lozada F. Prednisone and azathioprine in the treatment of patients with vesiculoerosive oral diseases. Oral Surgery 1981; 52 (3): 257.

56) Lozada-Nur F, Miranda C, Miliksi R. Double-blind clinical trial of 0.05% clobetasol proprionate ointment in orabase and 0.05%fluocinonide ointment in orabase in the treatment of patients with oral vesiculoerosive diseases. Oral Surg Oral Med Oral Pathol 1994; 77: 598-604.

57) Lozanda-Nur F, Gorsky M and Silverman S. Oral erythema multiforme: clinical observations and

treatment of 95 patients. Oral Surg Oral Med Oral Pathol 1989; 67: 36-40.

58) Lu S, Chen WJ, Eng HL. Dramatic response to levamisole and low-dose prednisolone in 23 patients with oral lichen planus - A 6-year prospective follow-up study. Oral Surg Oral Med Oral Pathol Oral Radiol Endod 1995; 80: 705-9.

59) Macphee IT, Sircus W, Farmer ED, et al. Use of steroids in treatment of aphthous ulceration. Br Med J 1968; 2: 147-149.

60) Mignogna MD, Muzio LL, Mignogna RE et al. Oral pemphigus: long term behagiour and clinical response to treatment with deflazacort in 16th case. J oral Pathol Med 2000;29: 145-52.

61) Miles DA, Bricker SL, Razmus TF, et al. Triamcinolone acetonide versus chlorhexidine for treatment of recurrent stomatitis. Oral Surg Oral Med Oral Pathol 1993; 75:397-402.

62) Miller CS, Dembo JB, Falace DA. Salivary cortisol response to dental treatment of varying stress. Oral Surg Oral Med Oral Pathol Oral Radiol Endod 1995; 79: 436-41.

63) Mosgaw SS, Schmelzeisen R, Frolich JC et al. Use of ibuprofen and methylprednisolone for the prevention of pain and swelling after removal of impacted third molars. J Oral Maxillofac Surg 1995; 53: 2-7.

64) Muhammad KJ, Lewis MAO, Crean SJ. Oral pemphigus vulgaris occurring during pregnancy. J Oral Pathol Med 2002; 31: 121-4.

65) Muralichar M, Raghavan MRV, Bailoor DN, et al. Bilateral Bell's palsy: current concepts in a etiology and treatment. Case report. Aust Dent J 1987; 32 (6) : 412 – 416.

66) Muzio LL, Valle AD, Mignogna MD, et al. The treatment of oral aphthous ulceration or erosive lichen planus with topical clobetasol propionate in three preparations: a clinical and pilot study on 54 patients. J Oral Pathol Med 2001; 30: 611-7.

67) Nasstrom K, Frosberg B, Petersson A et al. Narrowing of the dental pulp chamber in patients with renal diseases. Oral Surg. Oral Med. Oral Pathol 1985; 59: 242-246.

68) Neville BW, Damm DD, Allen CM et al. Viral Infections. In: Oral and Maxillofacial Pathology Saunders: Philadelphia 2nd ed. 2002: 213- 252.

69) Ogle OE, Ofodile F. The pharmacology of topical agents. Oral and Maxillofacial Surgery Clinics of North America 2002; 13: 119-130.

70) Papazian MR, Campbell JH, Nabi S. Management of Bell's palsy. J of Maxillofac surg 1993; 51: 661 – 665.

71) Paterson AJ, Lamey PJ, Nolan AL, et al. Pemphigus Vulgaris precipitated by glibenclamide therapy. J oral Pathol Med 1993; 22: 92-5.

72) Pedersen A, Klausen B. Glucocorticosteroids and oral medicine. J of oral path. 1984; 13: 1- 15.

73) Pimlott SJ, Walker DM. A controlled clinical trial of the efficacy of topically applied fluocinonide in the

treatment of recurrent aphthous ulceration. Br Dent J 1983; 154:174-177.

74) Plemons JM, Zachariah NY. Absorption of a topical steroid and evaluation of adrenal suppression in patients with erosive lichen planus. Oral Surg Oral Med Oral Pathol 1990; 69: 688-93.

75) Reith EJ, Ross MH.Endocrine System. In: Atlas of Descriptive Histology. WB Saunders Company; 3rd Edition 1980: 256-259

76) Rhodus NL, Janna B. Evaluation of a chemical cautery agent and an inflammatory ointment for the treatment of current aphthous stomatitis: a pilot study. Quintessccncc Int 1998; 29: 769-773.

77) Robinson JC, Lozada-Nur F, Frieden I. Oral pemphigus vulgaris a review of the literature and a report on the management of 12 cases. Oral Surg Oral Med Oral Pathol Oral Radiol Endod. 1997;84:349-55.

78) Ronald LTC, Butter CD, Vorono AA et al. Dosage effects of pulsed steroid therapy on serum cortisol levels in oral and maxillofacial surgery patients. Journal Maxillofac Surg 1993; 51: 750-753.

79) Satoskar RS, Bhandarkar DS, Ainapure SS et al. Adrenal cortical steroids. In: Pharmacology and pharmacotherapeutics. Popular prakashan Pvt. Ltd. Mumbai 15th ed.; 1997: 906- 926.

80) Schimmer BP, Parker KL.Adrenocorticotropic Hormone. In: Hurdman JG, Limbirl LE. Goodman and Gillman: The Pharmacological basis of therapeutics. Mc Gruehill – New York 2001: 1459- 1485.

81) Seymour RA, Walton JG. Pain control after third molar surgery. Int J Oral Surg. 1984; 13: 457-485.

82) Silva RG, Tolstunov L.Steroid – induced psychosis: report of case. Oral Maxillofac Surg 1995; 43: 183-186.

83) Silverman S, Gorksy M, Lozada- Nur F et al. A prospective study of findings and management in 214 patients with oral lichen planus. Oral surg oral med oral path 1991; 72: 665-70.

84) Sinnatamby CS. Suprarenal gland. In: Last's Anatomy – Regional and Functional Anatomy, Churchill Livingstone; 10th Edition 2001: 372.

85) Sirois D, Leigh JE, Sollecito TP. Oral pemphigus vulgaris preceding cutaneous lesions: recognition and diagnosis. JADA. 2000; 131: 1156-1160.

86) Sisk AL, Bonnington GJ. Evaluation of methylprednisolone and flurbiprofen for inhibition of the postoperative inflammatory response. Oral Surg Oral Med Oral Pathol 1985; 60: 137-145.

87) Sweeney CJ, Gilden DH. Ramsay Hunt syndrome. J Neurol Neurosurg Psychiatry 2001 Aug; 71(2): 149-54.

88) Takato T, Komuro Y, Yonehara Y. Giant hemangioma of the parotid gland associated with kasabach-merritt syndrome – a case report. J Oral Maillofac Surg 1993; 51: 425-428.

89) Terry BC, Jacoway JR. Management of central giant cell lesions. Oral and Maxillofacial surgery clinics of North America 1994; 6(3): 579-600.

90) Thomason JM, Girdler NM, Kendall-Taylor P et al. An investigation into the need for supplementary steroids in organ transplant patients undergoing gingival surgery. A double-blind, split-mouth, cross-over study. J Clin Periodontol 1999; 26: 577-582.

91) Thongprasom K, Laungjarmekorn L, Sererat T, et al. Relative efficacy of fluocinolone acetonide compared with triamcinolone acetonide in treatment of oral lichen planus. J Oral Pathol Med 1992; 21: 456-8.

92) Tjaderhane LS, Pajari UH, Ahola RH et al : Leaving the pulp chamber open for drainage has no effect on the complications of root canal therapy. Int Endo J 1995; 28: 82-85.

93) Tripati KD. Corticosteroids. In: Essentials of medical Pharmacology, Jaypee Brothers Medical Publishers: New Delhi 2004; 5th edition: 254- 265.

94) Vincent SD, Fotos PG, Baker KA et al. Oral lichen planus: The clinical, historical, and therapeutic features of 100 cases. Oral Surg Oral Med Oral Pathol 1990; 70: 165-71.

95) Vincent SD, Lilly GE. Clinical, historic, and therapeutic features of aphthous stomatitis. Oral Surg Oral Med Oral Pathol 1992; 74:79-86.

96) Voute BEA, Schulten EAJM, Langendijk PNJ et al. Fluocinonide in an adhesive base for treatment of oral lichen planus: a double-blind, placebo-controlled clinical study. Oral Surg Oral Med Oral Pathol 1993; 75: 181-5.

97) Wenneberg B, Kopp S, Grondahl HG et al. Long-term effect of intra-articular injections of a glucocorticosteroid into the TMJ: a clinical and radiographic 8-year follow-up. J Craniomandib Disord: Facial & Oral Pain 1991; 5: 11-18.

98) Wilcox JW, Hickory JE. Nonsurgical resolution of mucoceles. J Oral Surg 1979; 36: 478.

99) Wilson A, Schild HO, Modell W. Endocrinology. In: Applied physiology.Mosby Year Book: 13th ed. 1980: 527- 541.

100) Younai FS, Phelan JA. Oral mucositis with features of psoriasis – report of a case and review of the literature. Oral Surg Oral Med Oral Pathol Oral Radiol Endod 1997; 84: 61-7.

101) Zegarelli DJ. Multimodality steroid therapy of erosive and ulcerative oral lichen planus. J Oral Med 1983; 38 (3): 127-130.

***